Ultimate Chair Yoga for Seniors Over 60

An Illustrated Guide to Reduce the Risk of Falls with Easy 10-Minute Exercises to Increase Energy, Balance, and Flexibility

Roman Gurung

This is dedicated to my loving family – Ama, who is the inspiration behind this book, my amazing wife Rinku, and my incredible daughters Riannon, and particularly Rishona. Rishona's assistance with all the Chair Yoga asanas (poses) was invaluable to our illustrator for this book. Without everyone's love and support, this book would not have been published.

This is also dedicated to the loving memory of my late father, Hari Narain Singh Gurung, and my big brother, Rajesh (Roger) Gurung, who served and ultimately died for Canada on June 12, 1977. It's very rare a day goes by that they are not in my thoughts.

TABLE OF CONTENTS

INTRODUCTION

T hank you for choosing this book. I believe it is all you will need to enjoy your chair yoga experience.

While yoga often conjures images of incredibly fit people standing on their heads in fancy yoga classes, the actual beauty of yoga is that it can be adapted for anyone based on their personal abilities. Simple yet effective, chair yoga can be an excellent support for aging and specially-abled people, or anyone who wishes to start their yoga journey with the support of a chair.

With an increase in age comes many physical issues, be it aches and pains or life-threatening diseases. There are many reasons a person over 60 can feel hindered in their physical activities, including aging bones and muscles or loss of sensory sharpness, i.e., weak eyesight, hearing, etc. The risk of chronic diseases is also higher in older adults, but the most significant hindrance that these physical conditions bring is often mental. An increase in anxiety and fear is also common. Aging adults also often lose confidence in being able to manage many daily tasks or may feel their bodies do not allow them to do certain activities. An increased dependence on caregivers is another cause of fear, anxiety, and even depression. While the loss of physical independence can have a negative impact on a person's mental health, it also brings isolation as seniors are unable to participate in social events or family outings.

It would be callous to say that increased physical activity will solve most, if not all, of these problems because limited mobility brings about unique challenges for people beginning their exercise journey. Or even for active people who now find themselves restricted by their bodies, unable to exercise the way they did previously. Often, exercise designed for the general population does not apply to seniors. For much of the younger population, exercise is more about the aesthetics of their body. For people over 60, exercise is about maintaining and improving their mobility, managing pain and illnesses, and generally maintaining good health.

The apparent truth of fitness is that there is no one-size-fits-all. Seniors especially need exercises that not only help them maintain an appropriate weight but can help reduce muscle and joint stiffness. Something that can help them improve mobility and alleviate pain while also being low-impact and safe enough for them to perform by themselves. It needs to be something that doesn't require a heavy investment upfront, either on workouts or equipment, as seniors are often already retired and looking for budget-friendly options.

Adults over 80 are prone to falling, with an estimated 50% of people over 80 falling annually (Pain Doctor, 2019). However, chair yoga can significantly reduce this fear and risk of falling among the senior population. Continued practice of chair yoga can also provide relief from pain caused by osteoarthritis and reduce the hindrance caused by pain in everyday activities.

If you are struggling to get started with yoga or find yourself restricted because of your body, this book can help. Working your way through this book will bring you a step closer to managing chronic pain, feeling more flexible, and being as mobile as you can, whether you're 60 or 90. Independence will be within your control much longer if you take steps toward slowing down the natural aging process of your joints, muscles, and cognitive abilities. You'll enjoy those family gatherings, playdates with grandchildren, and visits with your friends. You'll decrease the risk of becoming dependent on those you love. You'll manage what you can to stay active as long as possible and embrace the golden part of your graceful years. The chair yoga techniques offered in this book can help you maintain an active and energetic life in the years to come.

I'm no stranger to the changes that come with aging. My mother is an 89-year-old lady who can still keep up with some of my fittest friends. She's feisty, healthier than most people her age, and she still drives her car, and competently at that! She's been through a lot in her long life and is the strongest person I know. She lives with me and my family; culturally speaking, as her son, it is my duty and obligation to care for her. As a family, we care for her together. My mom continues to be my inspiration.

However, her feistiness means she's pretty content with caring for herself and remaining independent. We've supported her every effort to remain independent and physically capable of joining us on many family outings. While she moves better than you'd expect, my mother is gradually slowing down as she nears her 90th birthday, at the time of this writing. Some people still can't believe how active she is, but her mobility, movements, and muscles aren't what they were. Fortunately, it didn't take much convincing. My mom is open to trying new things to help her remain as happy and healthy as possible for as long as possible. She began chair yoga after we researched the stretches and discussed the sequences with her healthcare provider. So, I've spent many hours reading about chair yoga and helping her find the sequences that work for mobility, strength, and balance.

My mother has come to love her daily practices and has made them part of her life. But it wasn't always straightforward with chair yoga; we didn't realize that in addition to chair yoga stretches, you also need the support of other gentle and low-impact exercises. Adding those along with simple dietary changes, breathwork, and mindfulness, she was able to transcend her daily practice and overall wellness. We came to realize how one's mind and body must work together. I didn't always understand the impact aging had on my mother until she improved physically but remained somewhat stuck mentally. Once we combined her efforts with mindfulness and breathwork that she practiced daily, she was rejuvenated with a new mind, heart, and body. Seeing the tremendous impact of chair yoga and other holistic practices on my mom, along with my team of researchers, we combined all of our discoveries and wisdom into this comprehensive guide.

The first chapter of the book focuses on preparing oneself for the practice. We look at why chair yoga is the best option for you and understand the nuances of what it really is and its benefits. In the second chapter, we look at the necessary preparations to make before attempting chair yoga to gain maximum benefits from the exercises. We discuss various techniques to safely warm up the body before exercise, as well as cool-down stretches. We also go over other preparatory details about the space, choosing the right chair, and what else to prepare for an optimal exercise session. In chapter three, the focus is on food, and we talk about a supportive diet that you can maintain along with the chair yoga exercises to maintain good health.

Often, certain foods that we ate in our younger days become detrimental to our health as we age. We discuss all those foods and why they are no longer beneficial for our bodies at an older age. It is important to remember that diet is subjective, and often, genetics tend to play a role in what foods are more suited for our bodies. Any new diets should always be introduced with the guidance of healthcare professionals. The chapter after that is about exploring the mind-body connection. The mental health of seniors is something that is often overlooked. We dive deeper into improving older adults' mental and cognitive states as this can greatly affect their physical health and the benefits they experience with chair yoga in both specific and physical exercises in general.

In the second half of the book, we get into the meat and potatoes of chair yoga and supportive exercises. We start with chapter five, where we discuss in-depth supportive cardio that helps to maintain heart health, as well as various breathing exercises to improve lung capacity and lung function. Chapter 6 introduces the first of the three sequences of chair yoga practices. It describes the issues that will be addressed by following the described sequence and then goes on to explain the first ten-minute chair yoga sequence. Chapter 7 is all about the second chair yoga sequence, which is important for maintaining muscle mass while strengthening the muscle fibers as we age. We also discuss aspects of muscle loss and why muscle strength becomes more relevant as we age.

The final chapter discusses joint and chronic pain issues and describes the final chair yoga sequence, which is specially focused on pain management. With this book, we hope we have provided a comprehensive guide on how to maintain or improve the quality of life for an aging population in a simple yet effective manner.

CHAPTER 1

What Makes Chair Yoga Worth Your Time?

Yoga is one of the most popular methods of exercise today. Every morning, you can find people at any local park, twisted like a pretzel. You might see this and believe that this is all yoga is, which essentially translates to "I can't do this." If that is the case, you would be surprised to know that over 14 million North Americans above 50 years old practice various forms of yoga (Baiera, 2021). And 87% of senior yogis report reduced pain and stiffness in muscles and joints. But how? That is because the greatest thing about yoga is the different ways that it can be practiced. Yoga practices include *Vinyasa, Ashtanga, Bikram, Hatha*, and power yoga. Among these is chair yoga, one of the more senior-friendly ways of practicing yoga. So before we start doing the yoga exercises, let's understand what exactly chair yoga is.

What Is Chair Yoga?

As the name suggests, chair yoga is doing yoga on a chair. It is based on the poses used in traditional yoga, which people started practicing over 5,000 years ago. It is easy to replicate most of the traditional poses so that they can be practiced in a seated position. This makes chair yoga suitable and enjoyable for individuals at all experience levels, including seniors. Because of the way the exercises are designed it has become the latest fad among seniors. The chair modification enables them to do most of the traditional yoga exercises in an easier version while gaining similar benefits.

In 1982, yoga therapist Lakshmi Voelker developed chair yoga with a specific purpose in mind (Rucki, 2022). By utilizing a chair for support, stability, and enhanced mobility, chair yoga could help aging individuals or those with physical limitations get the same benefits as those who practiced traditional yoga. Chair yoga offers real advantages for those managing chronic pain, carpal tunnel syndrome, osteoporosis, multiple sclerosis (MS), and a range of other chronic conditions. It also provides a highly effective alternative for people of all ages who are recovering from surgery or injuries that limit their ability to engage in traditional yoga practice.

A natural question that comes up is, how do I know if chair yoga is for me? The short answer is that chair yoga is for everyone. Chair yoga is for anyone who finds traditional yoga to be too advanced or difficult for them to perform in their current situation. Anyone who wishes to do yoga with the support of a chair can do so. However, chair yoga is more ideal for certain groups than others. Some of these groups are:

- People 65 and older: This group can especially benefit from chair yoga as it is a low-impact way to maintain health and slow down the aging process. It is also a safer alternative to many other forms of exercise as there is a reduced risk of falling or other injuries.

- People with chronic health conditions: A 2019 study published in the American Journal of Alzheimer's Disease and Other Dementias suggests that chair yoga can be beneficial for people suffering from dementia. There is growing research on the benefits of chair yoga on chronic diseases and related pain management such as arthritis and diabetes. This can make chair yoga a wonderful option for people with chronic diseases.

- People with limited mobility: People with certain physical impairments, for example, patients suffering from MS or spinal cord injuries benefit from chair yoga. Even people with temporary impairments like major surgeries or injuries can use chair yoga for exercise and rehabilitation.

- People who work in an office: People who are required to spend a lot of time in an office, or mostly in a seated position can benefit from stretches and exercises that they can perform from the comfort of their chair. This group of people is more susceptible to back pain, neck and shoulder pain, and mental stressors. Chair yoga can help them improve both their physical and mental states without having to leave their office.

While these are some of the groups that can leverage chair yoga, everyone can enjoy the benefits. However, it is important to remember that any new exercise routine should only be incorporated with the advice of a healthcare professional.

Particularly for seniors with existing health conditions, special care should be taken so that the exercise doesn't interfere with the doctor's recommended lifestyle. Otherwise, chair yoga can be practiced anywhere between two to three times per week for seniors over 65. But if that sounds like a lot, you can always start with the number of days that you are comfortable with and build up from there.

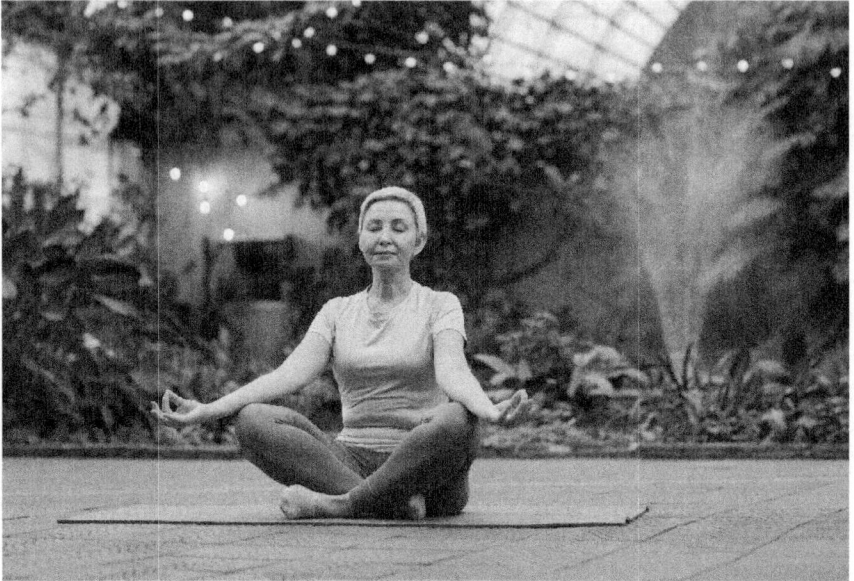

Benefits of Chair Yoga

Chair yoga, like all exercise routines, helps improve the physical fitness of the body. It has a number of other benefits for your overall lifestyle as well. Let's look at some of the most common benefits of chair yoga:

- Flexibility and balance. Yoga is already known for improving flexibility and balance, with chair yoga, seniors can also experience an improvement in their flexibility. According to a study done in 2010 by Schmid et al., seniors who practiced chair-based yoga practices twice a week for twelve weeks witnessed increased lower body flexibility and balance.

- Strength. Another benefit of chair yoga is an improvement in muscle tone and strength. Increased strength reduces the risk of falls, and improved muscle tone makes you more resilient to injuries.

- Improved self-awareness. Chair yoga often involves seamless and smooth movements; this, combined with the focus required to get to and from each posture, creates a heightened awareness of the space around us and, as a result, also of ourselves.

- Reduced stress. Because of the nature of movements and yogic exercises, it can help you develop an increase in awareness and mindfulness. A natural side effect of this is a reduction in overall stress by providing relaxation and mental clarity.

- Pain management skills. Any exercise releases natural painkillers in the form of endorphins. As you strengthen your muscles and bones, the pain is not only reduced, but your pain endurance and management capabilities also increase.

- Improved sleep. Relaxation, mindfulness, and exercise are known to improve the quality of your sleep. It induces deeper sleep, which provides the body with the necessary rest and restoration to function in the best way possible.

- Helps manage chronic conditions. Generally, as yoga balances out your system, it can also help to manage chronic conditions like blood pressure, sugar levels, etc. In fact, a small 2016 pilot study by Park et al. concluded that seniors practicing yoga regularly for three months experienced an improvement in their diabetes-related conditions.

- Boost mood and mental well-being. The mindfulness and breathwork aspect of yoga can provide a mental balance, which can help to alleviate symptoms of depression, panic attacks, and anxiety. These same benefits extend to chair yoga as well.

- Reduced fear of falling. A 2012 study by Galantino et al. suggests that as seniors gain strength and balance, they have a decreased fear of falling and an increase in confidence and independence in leaving their residence and partaking in more overall activity.

- Spiritualism and Mindfulness. A 2018 study by Kertapati et al. concluded that the use of chair yoga with spiritual intervention is a useful preventive measure against a functional decline in older adults.

All seniors can gain these benefits by practicing chair yoga regularly. The benefits specific to seniors suffering from osteoarthritis are significant, these include:

- Joint flexibility. Numerous studies suggest that seniors with osteoarthritis experience improved flexibility in their joints after a few weeks of practicing chair yoga (Park et al., 2014).

- Mobility and gait speed (how long it takes someone to travel a given distance). While this is true for everyone practicing chair yoga, this benefit is especially significant for seniors suffering from osteoarthritis as they experience the most impairment in mobility due to their condition.

- Functional fitness. Chair yoga can help to improve functional fitness and ease of daily activities for seniors who have knee osteoarthritis.

While numerous, the above-mentioned benefits are not exhaustive, and the impact chair yoga can have on your quality of life is second to none. Despite all this, many people are reluctant to start practicing chair yoga because of the misconceptions about this practice. In the next section, we bust some common myths about chair yoga.

Myths About Chair Yoga

- **Chair Yoga isn't real exercise.** This is possibly the most common myth about yoga overall. We often associate yoga with slow, controlled movements. While these types of movements are common in yoga, that is not all yoga. There are fast-paced and difficult movements and poses that require not just balance and flexibility but also strength and agility. Vinyasa or Ashtanga yoga are some examples of this type of yoga.

- **You are too old**. Another common myth among seniors is that you are too old to practice yoga. And that is simply not true. with the number of yoga

7

variations available, and especially with chair yoga, there is something for everybody!

- **It's only for women**. This common misconception is quite ironic because, in ancient India, it was men who primarily practiced and taught yoga. Because of its connection to spirituality, the Western world started associating it with women. But just as spirituality is for both men and women, so is yoga.

- **Chair yoga can't help you lose weight**. Any form of exercise, done regularly and with a supportive diet, can help you lose weight. The same is true for chair yoga. In fact, it might be one of the safest ways to lose weight, with the least risk of injury.

- **You can't do chair yoga when you're in pain**. In reality, the reverse is true. Doing yoga can actually help relieve pain and the body stretches and relaxes, often reducing muscle tension and providing relief.

- **Chair yoga is only for seniors**. While popular among seniors, chair yoga is for anyone who finds getting down on a mat challenging for any reason. Chair yoga helps to improve accessibility for those who find themselves unable to try traditional yoga.

- **You simply stretch out in a chair**. Some people think you can just doze off on a chair and call it chair yoga. If you believe that is all chair yoga is, you are in for a surprise. There are a variety of exercises that you can do in chair yoga, either sitting on the chair or using it for support.

- **It is the easiest form of yoga**. Chair yoga may be one of the most convenient ways of doing yoga, but that doesn't mean it is easy. Because it can be adjusted to your level, you can make it as easy or as difficult as you like.

- **You need a special chair**. There are certain requirements for a chair to be optimal for usage with chair yoga. you don't really need a "special" chair to practice chair yoga.

- **Any chair works.** Again, while most chairs would work well for chair yoga, there are certain features a chair should have for the best results.

What About Results?

We all want an independent and pain-free life where we can participate fully and without worrying about ourselves or others. In fact, for most of us, that is the motivation for picking up this book. So, it is natural to wonder if and when you will see results. If you practice chair yoga three times a week for four weeks, you may begin to see results. There will not be drastic changes, but you might experience simpler things like ease of daily activities and an improved mood. To see a significant change in your physical condition, like reduced pain or weight loss, it might take longer, anywhere from twelve weeks or more but it could be less, too. The key is not to give up. The speed of physical improvements is subjective and will vary from person to person. It may be faster for some and slower for others, but if you follow the right diet and engage in mindfulness along with a disciplined practice of

9

chair yoga, you will definitely experience all the benefits and more.

Wisdom is not a product of schooling but a lifelong attempt to acquire it.

— Albert Einstein

You are never too old to learn something new. Einstein believed wisdom came from constantly learning new things. Educating yourself about why chair yoga works for you also helps you obtain a growth mindset. You also won't feel confident in your chair yoga practice without understanding the facts. With the facts already covered, let's move away from the boring informational things and start preparing for chair yoga benefits!

CHAPTER 2

Preparation Makes Perfect Sense

What would you usually do when you have to take an exam? You prepare for it. You study and ensure you have the correct examination pass and the necessary equipment to complete it, whether it is writing material or your laptop. In the same way, chair yoga tests your joints, abilities, muscles, and balance. So, it is crucial to do proper preparation before attempting chair yoga. Warming up is essential, whether running a mile or doing a 10-minute chair yoga sequence. A total warm-up of 3-5 minutes can save you from stiffer or more achy joints tomorrow.

Similarly, a proper cool-down stretch can ensure that you do not experience extra aches due to muscle soreness. Soreness often happens if we use our normally sedentary muscles after a long time. Let's guide you in preparing for sequences and ensuring your safety before you get to the chair yoga poses.

Preparing Your Space

Preparing your space can sound very simple, but there are many aspects to it. You have to consider not just the chair you are planning to use but any other equipment you might need for support, what you should wear, and many other small but essential things. Let's take a look at what you can do to maintain an optimal space for chair yoga practice.

Clearing the Space

It is important to have some room around the chair so that you can perform all the movements comfortably without hindrance. It helps in case you experience dizziness or blacking out during the exercise. In the eventuality that you are about to fall, a clear space can ensure you don't hit sharp objects or sustain additional injuries. While these situations are uncommon, it is better to be prepared for the worst when we venture into a new physical activity. In case you experience dizziness or are close to blacking out, stop doing what you were doing, sit comfortably, and focus on your breathing. If this situation arises due to existing medical conditions, please follow the guidance of your healthcare provider.

What to Wear?

When attempting chair yoga, one should wear comfortable, moderately close-fitting athletic clothing. It helps you to avoid overheating while keeping your joints and muscles supported. It also means the clothes don't catch on objects, helping to prevent any unexpected falls. Many people prefer to wear shoes while doing chair yoga. If shoes can be supportive or you are doing it in a place with cold floors, you can definitely wear them. But wearing shoes is not mandatory for the practice.

Choosing Your Chair

One of the most critical aspects of chair yoga, other than actually practicing it, is choosing the right chair. You may think, "A chair is a chair," What is so special about it? But when practicing yoga on a chair, there are many nuances that could seriously affect your experience of the practice and even your safety while performing it. So, what are some of the things you should look for when choosing a chair? Let's explore:

- **Height**. Choose a chair that, when you sit on it, your feet reach the ground comfortably. Ensure that your feet are flat on the ground for maximum stability.

- **The seat of the chair**. A big feature to look out for is that the seat is completely flat. Also, ensure that it is level from front to back and side to side. A flat and level seat is the most supportive for the different chair yoga postures.

- **Sturdiness**. Saying that a chair should be sturdy is an understatement. But you need to ensure that when you move around in the chair, lean back, or move to the side, it doesn't tip because of the weight distribution. If that is happening on the chair, then it is not safe for chair yoga.

- **Chair back**. Ensure that the back is comfortable and supportive for you and is not causing hindrance with movement.

- **Arms**. You might think a chair with arms is unsuitable for yoga, but that is not entirely true. Seniors who need support for sitting down or getting up can use a chair with arms. Sure, it will restrict some movements, but it is still possible to practice chair yoga if you need chair arms for support. So, whether you use a chair with or without arms is dependent on your situation. Some of the types of chairs that would work well for chair yoga are below.

Standard Chair

Most standard kitchen or desk chairs work well for chair yoga. A folding metal chair or a wooden kitchen chair would also work fine. You only need to ensure that the criteria mentioned above are fulfilled, especially concerning the height and stability of the chair. As long as the key criteria are met, any chair available in your home would work well.

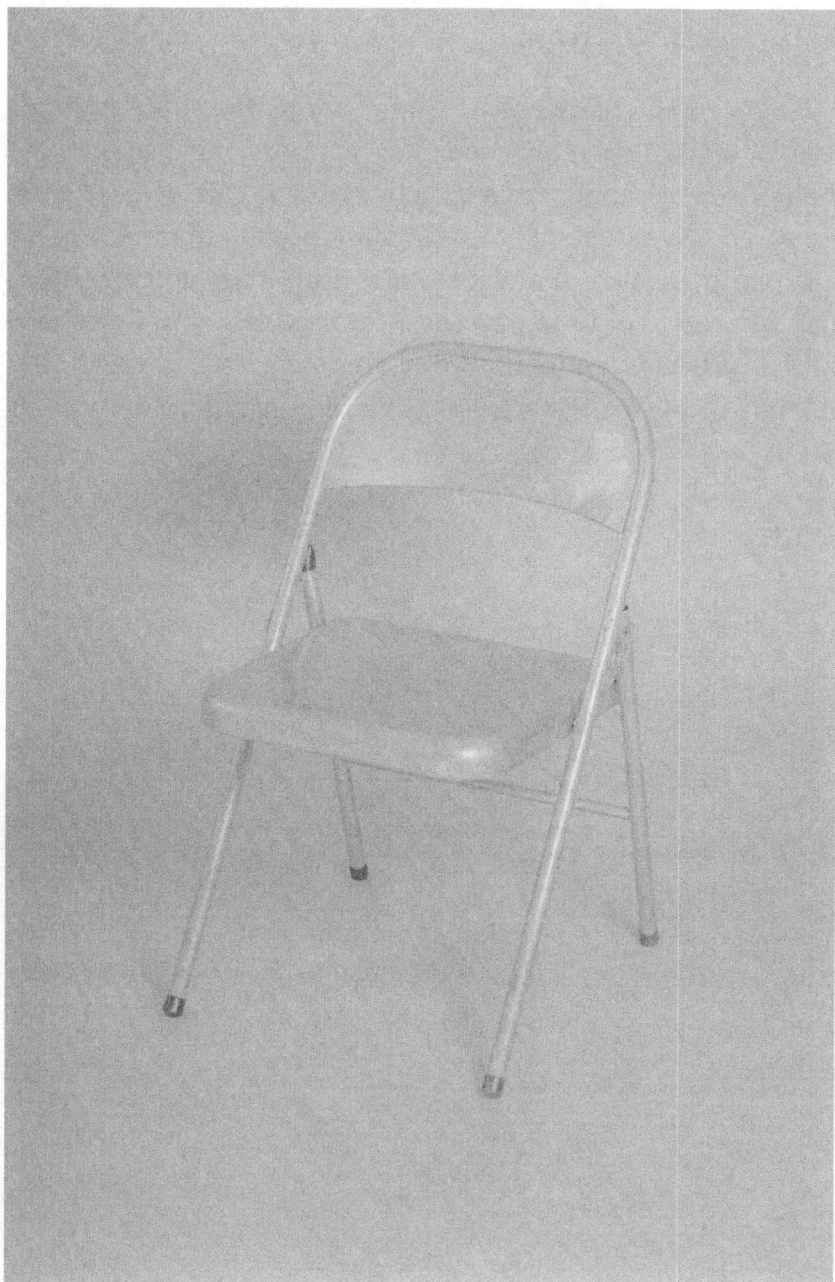

Balance Ball Chair

Balance ball chairs are becoming more and more popular because of their postural benefits. It is possible to use such a chair for your chair yoga practice and it can give you an increased advantage of strengthening your core muscles and improving posture. However, it is important to remember that stability should not be compromised in using this chair. If it has wheels, ensure that they are locked or placed so that it doesn't move. Always ensure that the key criteria for a chair are always fulfilled.

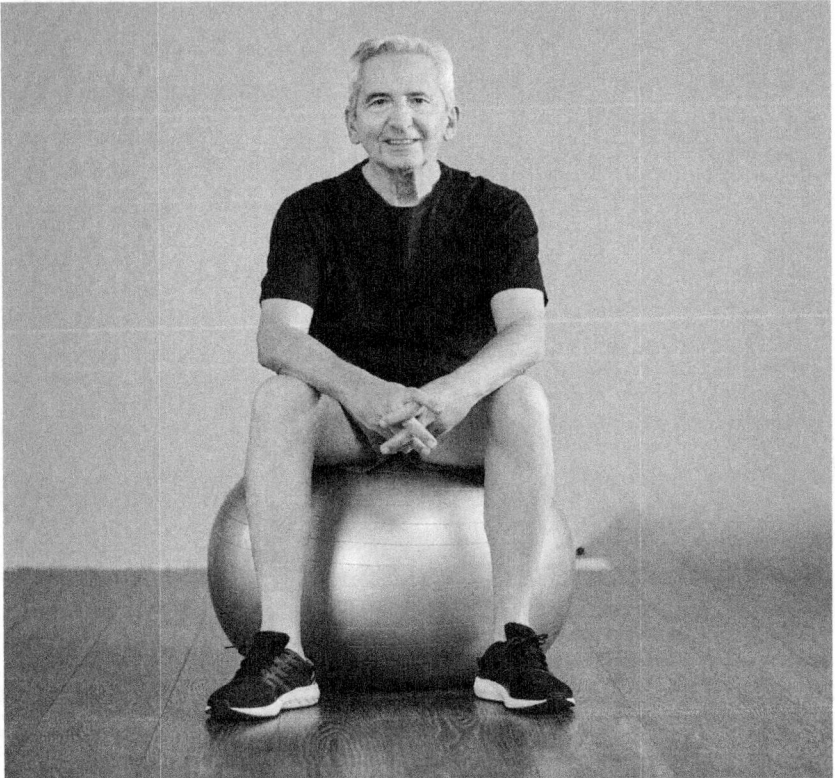

Office Chair

An office chair can be another handy option if you want to practice chair yoga in your office. Even normal desk chairs work fine. Again, you might want to be careful if the chair has wheels and armrests and ensure that the chair provides the necessary stability. Making sure that the essential criteria are attained in a chair is a sure-fire way to determine whether the chair is suitable for your yoga practice.

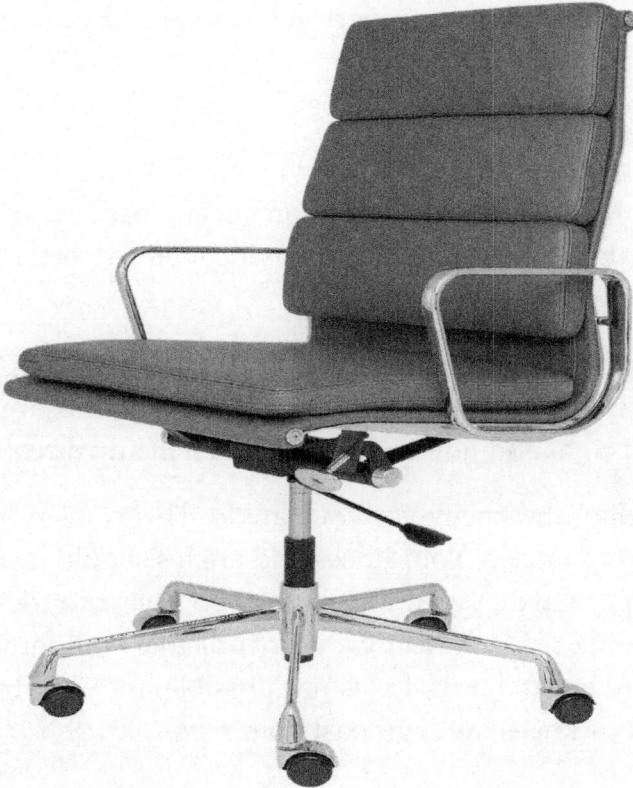

Safety Precautions

Now that we have the basics of preparation down, let's look at some of the safety precautions you should take when performing chair yoga. We will also go over certain special precautions you should take if you are struggling with issues like osteoarthritis and hypertension.

Basic Precautions for Chair Yoga

- Maintain focus on how your body feels during the practice. Yoga is a very mindful practice on its own, but deliberate attention to your body will help you identify the difference between discomfort and pain.

- Breathe consciously but with ease. As you continue to inhale and exhale at an even pace your body automatically relaxes, allowing you to perform yoga better.

- Sit upright. You don't have to sit ramrod straight or in an unnatural manner, but ensure that you are sitting upright and not leaning too much in any direction.

- Align the knee over your ankle. This is a key rule for any exercise. Your knees and ankles should be aligned in a way that your knees don't go past your toes at any point. A perfectly perpendicular alignment is preferred, but if this is not possible, try your best that your knees don't go past your toes.

- Keep your feet flat on the floor. This is important for stability and balance as you perform chair yoga. Unless an exercise explicitly needs your foot to be raised off the ground, keep your feet flat or as close to flat as possible.

- Avoid straining. Make sure to perform the exercises only to a level of discomfort and not pain. As mentioned in the first point, keep focus and try to understand your body's signals to avoid straining yourself too much and causing injuries.

- Avoid jerking and bouncing. Try to keep all your movements smooth and gradual. Do not go abruptly from one movement to another as sudden, jerky movements might cause straining or injury to your muscles and joints.

I Have Osteoarthritis/Osteoporosis/Osteopenia

If you have osteoarthritis, spinal degeneration, or any other back issues, please make sure to avoid any stretches that put pressure on sensitive or problem areas. In this case, you can replace stretches with breathing techniques when the sequences call for bending forward or doing specific exercises that may hurt your back further.

Similarly, for people suffering from osteoporosis or osteopenia, extra care should be taken to avoid back injuries. Since these conditions make your bones weaker, there is a higher possibility of fractures. Two exercises in particular that should be avoided are spine flexion, or bending forward, and spine rotation, or twisting.

If you take these few precautions, you should be able to perform all other exercises comfortably.

I Have Hypertension

Those with high blood pressure will have to follow certain precautions to ensure a safe practice. Avoid all types of inversions and any exercise where the head is below the heart, try to use modifications instead. Gentler twists and stretches should be included in the practice and any abrupt movements should be avoided. This will help you to avoid an unnecessary rise in blood pressure as well as dizziness or light-headedness.

As a general rule when practicing chair yoga, it is best to follow the safety precautions and modify any exercises as necessary for your fitness levels. Remain mindful during the practice and in case of extreme pain and discomfort, stop the practice. Remember to consult with your healthcare professional before starting any new exercise routine.

Preparing Yourself

Oftentimes we do a lot to prepare everything else but forget to prepare ourselves for the task that we are about to perform. The same can be true for chair yoga. So, in this section, we are going to discuss everything you can do to prepare your body and mind for chair yoga exercises. These tips are similar to the instructions you might receive from an instructor at the beginning of a live session. So, many of these might sound familiar, but it is always good to refresh these instructions before practice for a safe, engaging, and productive yoga session.

Preparing Your Body

Here are some steps you can take to prepare your body for your practice.

- **Keep your sessions short and simple**. Keeping your practice simple will help you feel safe and confident while performing yoga. Do not involve unnecessarily complex movements until you feel ready for it. Instead of trying to perfect each pose, try instead to ensure that you are involving the right muscle groups and you are feeling the stretch or discomfort at the right spots. This will help you avoid injuries and extract maximum advantage from the practice.

- **Consider your limitations**. Be mindful of any injuries or degenerative disorders that may prevent certain stretches. Be conscious of them before practice, and avoid any stretches that extend discomfort to pain. Instead, use modifications or support while performing the exercise or replace the stretch with a mindful breathing technique.

- **Add more dynamic movements**. As you get more comfortable with the practice, you can progressively add dynamic movements. Adding such movements can reduce stiffness as well as improve blood circulation in your limbs.

- **Add props.** You can add props to support your chair yoga practice or even make it more challenging. Some of the commonly used props are:

    o **Yoga blocks.** An example of using yoga blocks can be if you are having trouble planting your feet on the floor in a stable manner. You can use yoga blocks underneath your feet to provide a raised floor to rest your feet on stably.

- o **Cushions.** You can use cushions if you have longer legs that are slanting when you sit down. If this is the case, you can put a cushion on your chair and sit on it to raise yourself higher so that your legs are perfectly parallel to the floor and your pelvis and knees are on the same plane.

- o **Straps.** These help students get deeper into poses or perform poses that they do not have the range of motion to perform.

- **End with Savasana or corpse pose**. Savasana is a common *yogasana* used for cool-down. In this pose, you lie down either on the floor or a relatively firm surface, close your eyes and relax your body focusing on your breath. Doing savasana at the end of your practice helps both the mind and the body to rest, digest, and become calm. During this time we can go back and observe any thoughts and feelings that might have come up during the class. Savasana is normally done lying down but there are modifications to do it on the chair as well.

- **Always use warm-up and cool-down sequences**. Both warming up and cooling down the body are extremely important to avoid injuries and pain in your muscles and joints.

Preparing Your Mind

Preparing yourself mentally can sometimes be much more important than any physical preparation. There is a saying that all battles are first won or lost in the mind. This implies that your thoughts and mindset have great power to influence the outcome of anything that you do. This being said, preparing your mind becomes the most imperative step. So, let's take a look at what are some of the things we can do for this.

- Set intentions. Setting an intention for a session can help you maintain focus throughout the session and you can keep coming back to it periodically to center yourself during the practice. Some examples of simple intentions that you can set are:

  o Physical intentions, for example, focusing on a specific part of the body, such as opening up the hips or shoulders, or strengthening your knees.

  o Energetic intentions, for example, producing a specific energetic effect, such as lifting the energy in the room.

  o Emotional intentions, for example, cultivating or maintaining a certain attitude or emotion, such as happiness or gratitude.

  o Theme-based intentions, such as setting an intention related to a specific theme or topic — for example, the season you're in, or something like self-care or gaining confidence.

- **Mindfulness**. While yoga naturally guides us to become more peaceful and mindful, it is helpful to be conscious of your mind while practicing yoga. Keeping your mind with the smooth yoga movements in the present moment can help you cultivate a generally meditative mind. Incorporating more breathing techniques and meditative practices can also help you with anxiety and depression.

- **Motivation and a positive mindset**. Motivation is easy to gain and just as easy to lose. Keeping a positive attitude when approaching chair yoga can make all the difference in your practice. Starting something new can be daunting, but if you approach it with the mindset of experimentation and playfulness, you can make a seemingly difficult task easy. Maintaining this positive attitude and discipline is also key because only if you continue to practice with sincerity will you be able to maintain this attitude long-term.

- **Breathing techniques**. Breathing exercises or *pranayama* is another important step to prepare your mind and body. As we do various breathing techniques with ease and continuity, it naturally relaxes our body and puts our mind at ease. Diaphragmatic breathing — breathing deeply from the stomach — is a breathing practice that causes the spine to extend and the small intercostal muscles below the ribs to contract. This increases the oxygen in your lungs and improves blood circulation while reducing the tension in your body at the same time. This means that the blood is better oxygenated, allowing the body to function at a higher level.

Let's Warm-Up Together

We have looked at preparation at length. Now we finally get to move ourselves! Starting with a warm-up and cool-down routine. This is a basic stretch that can be applicable to most sequences; as you advance in your chair yoga practice, you can add other, more specific warm-up stretches to this routine to suit your needs.

To start with, sit comfortably on the chair with your back straight and your spine slightly stretched. Focusing on your breath continue to breathe deeply to center yourself. Next, perform these stretches to open up your muscles and joints.

1. LATERAL STRETCH

Breathe in and extend your right arm all the way up, making sure to keep your shoulder away from your ear, and your neck relaxed. As you breathe out, take a lateral stretch by bending towards the left. Press your right thigh down; you may use your left hand, if needed, for a deeper stretch. Stay here for a few breaths, and with an exhalation come back to the center, bringing your right arm down. Repeat on the other side.

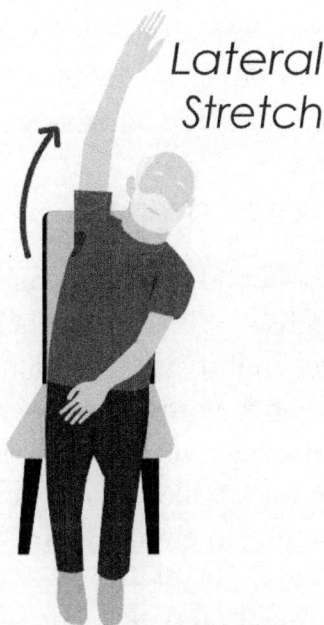

Lateral Stretch

2. TWISTING

Before twisting, place your right hand on the seat at the back of the chair. Breathe in, and as you exhale, twist your torso to the left. Keep your shoulders relaxed, and reach out with the left hand to hold the right side of the chair. Hold the twist and breathe deeply from the abdomen. Remain in the stretch as long as it is comfortable, taking

Twisting

steady breaths throughout. To get out of the pose, as you let go of the chair, inhale deeply, and come back to the center. Repeat on the other side.

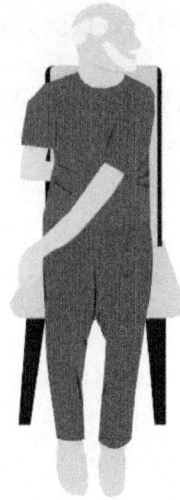

3. CAT-COW POSE

Place your palms on your thighs. With an inhalation, press lightly into the palms and hunch your upper back, bringing your ribs inside, taking a hollow body position. Bring your chin to your chest as if you want to go within yourself. Breathe out as you come back to the neutral position.

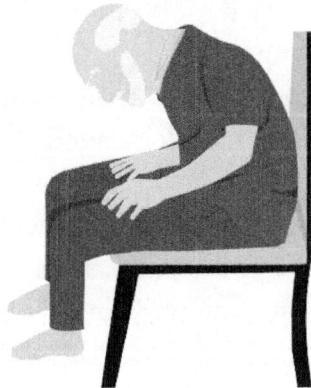

Cat-Cow Pose

You can repeat these exercises a few times as needed to fully relax and open up the muscles and joints. These same exercises can be used when cooling down as well.

Some additional movements you can add to this routine, as needed, are:

NECK ROLLS

To stretch the muscles on your neck and shoulders, you can perform neck rolls as part of the warm-up. Follow the steps below:

1. Take a deep breath in, and, as you exhale, bend your head towards your right shoulder by bringing your right ear closer to it. Make sure to keep your left shoulder down; do not let it tilt or move in the direction of your ear. Keep this pose for a few seconds.

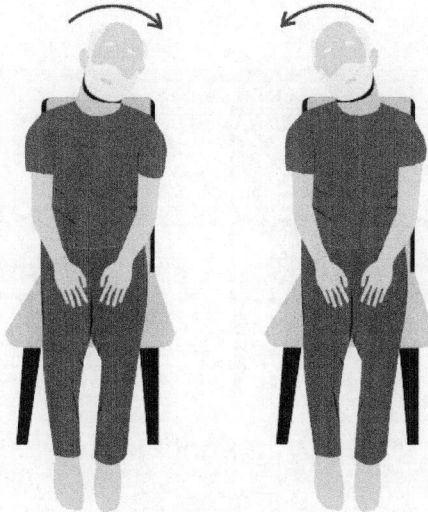

Neck Rolls

2. Inhale and bring your neck back to the center.

3. Inhale, and, as you are exhaling, bend your head towards your left shoulder by bringing your left ear closer to it. Remain here for a few seconds.

4. Inhale and come back to the center. Repeat this exercise for a few rounds on both sides.

It may seem like a lot of steps for a simple exercise, but the combination of breathing and movement is important, so try to follow the instructions closely.

FOOT FLEXING

Doing foot flexions can ensure that your ankle and calf muscles are properly stretched. Follow the steps below to perform proper stretching:

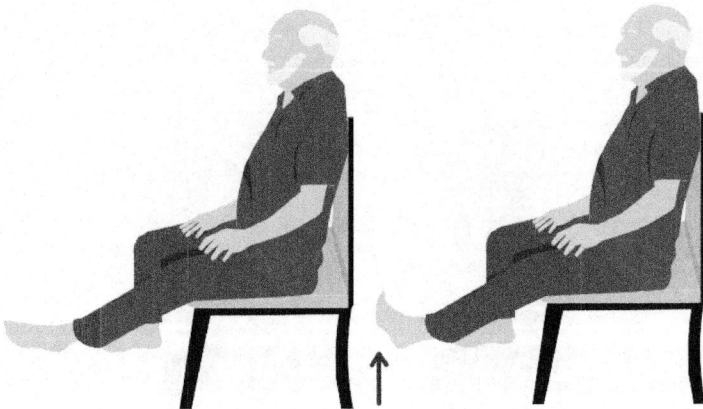

Foot Flexing

1. Inhale and raise your left leg to about a 40-degree angle, while keeping your right foot comfortably on the floor.

2. Inhale and stretch your left ankle, flexing your left foot and toes up and down while keeping the leg at 40 degrees.

3. Do this movement about 10 times and then pause. Keep your foot in the air for a few breaths, feeling the stretch at the Achilles tendon.

4. Release your left leg and repeat the same stretches 10 times on the right leg.

Take care of your body. It's the only place you have to live.

—Jim Rohn

Caring for your body means you can't dive head-first into an exercise routine, even if it only lasts 10 minutes. You must care for your body's needs, warm up, cool down, and practice safety in every step while you prepare to practice chair yoga. This truly is the only place you have to live. Don't damage it before you start. Once you prepare everything and familiarize yourself with the warm-up routines, you can dive into the nutritional tips you need to support your chair yoga workouts.

CHAPTER 3

What You Eat Can Support a Daily Chair Yoga Practice

I f you have enough exposure to the health and fitness industry you might have seen it coming, but others might be wondering what eating has to do with yoga. Sure, people say muscles are made in the kitchen, but we aren't trying to do that. So then, why a discussion on food? Any fitness professional who knows what they are talking about will never let you go without a lecture on food. It really is that big a part of our health and fitness.

What you eat can affect not only the weight on your scale or what you see in the mirror—food can affect our thoughts, actions, and behaviors. So, when venturing into a new health regimen, it only makes sense to revisit what you are eating and how it has been serving you. We all know how proteins can affect our muscle composition and strength. Similarly eating or avoiding certain foods can affect our flexibility, inflammation levels, and agility levels, among other abilities. What you eat or avoid can help your chair yoga routine. In addition, if weight gain has been a concern, it may help you lose a few pounds.

A shift to a sedentary lifestyle from a more active one as we age can also play with weight. Either way, some foods are better in our prime years, while we should stay as far away as possible from other foods. An example of this is red meat, one of the most common inflammatory foods you can eat. Inflammation won't help you lose weight or move easily as you age. Instead, you'll probably need some tips and diet tricks to help keep inflammation at bay while practicing daily chair yoga, one of which is ironically, consuming protein.

Some General Guidelines

In the later sections, we look at specific foods and their properties that may help or hinder our chair yoga practice and overall well-being. But first, we go through some general guidelines to use what we eat as a tool for our growth.

Eating Whole Foods

Integrating more whole foods into your diet can improve your digestion and your gut health. Consuming whole foods, such as fruits, vegetables, seeds, nuts, poultry, fish, legumes, and grains, provides vital nutrients essential for maintaining a healthy weight. Having more whole foods in your diet can also help with weight loss.

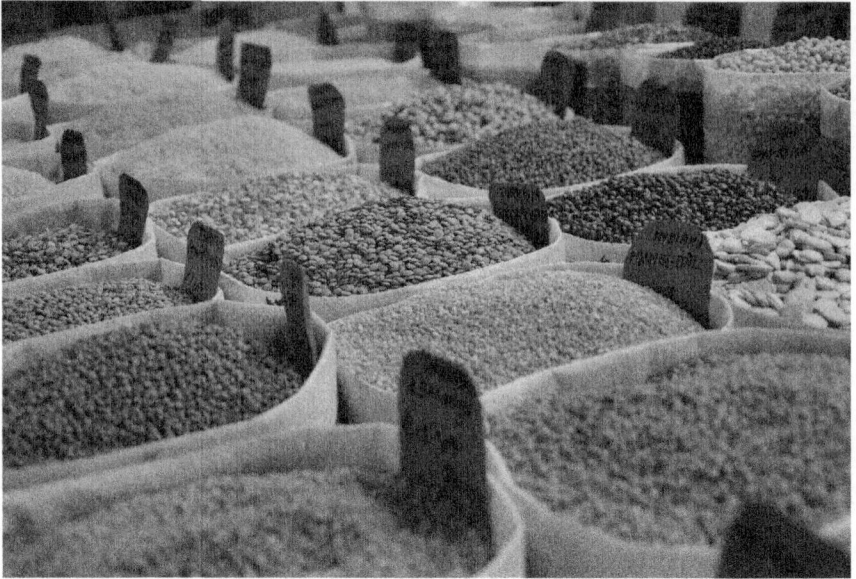

Timing Your Meals

While it is not necessary to stick to meal times by the hour, having dinner earlier in the night is known to have many benefits. It can assist you by shedding excess weight and keeping it off. It can also reduce the likelihood of metabolic syndrome, which is a group of conditions including high blood sugar and excess belly fat. Generally speaking, having an early dinner means your body gets more time to digest the food before you sleep and your bodily functions slow down. This results in better digestion and better absorption of nutrients, making the same food provide more benefits and helping you feel lighter at the same time.

Adding More Produce to Your Diet

Fruits and vegetables are packed with nutrients that are critical to your health. Adding them to your diet is a simple, but effective way to drop excess weight.

Several studies have shown that a higher consumption of vegetables and fruits can help in reducing body weight, and waist circumference, particularly in dropping excess fat (Yu et. al., 2018). When introducing fruits and vegetables into your diet, take care in case there is anything you know or suspect you could be allergic to. If such concerns exist, only introduce more fruits and veggies to your diet after consulting a medical professional.

Intermittent Fasting

Intermittent fasting involves only eating within a set amount of hours in the day and fasting for the rest. Several studies have shown that increasing the intake of vegetables and fruits can contribute to weight loss and reductions in waist circumference with insulin resistance, which is linked to chronic illnesses like diabetes and hormonal imbalances like polycystic ovarian syndrome (PCOS) in women (Yuan et. al., 2022). Introducing this fasting practice to your lifestyle can help with weight loss, support your yoga practice and, at the same time, reduce the impact of chronic illnesses.

Staying Hydrated

Hydration can sometimes be a tricky concept. We often drink something or the other throughout the day that makes us feel like we are sufficiently hydrated. But what we are drinking matters more than we think. Sweetened coffee beverages, soda, juices, sports drinks, pre-made smoothies, and other drinks, while liquid, do little in terms of hydrating the body. Water is the best possible way to hydrate our bodies. Any plain, potable water will do the trick better than anything else. If you don't like the taste, you can have herbal teas but avoid any other artificially sweetened drinks, especially those containing high-fructose corn syrup.

Choosing the Right Supplements

With time, there has been a gradual decline in the amount of nutrients that even naturally occurring foods contain. Along with that, as you grow older your ability to absorb nutrients decreases. A combination of these factors means there is a higher risk of nutrient deficiencies as we age. To counter this, we should include the right supplements in our diet. Deficiencies in B vitamins like B12 can lead to mood disturbances, cause fatigue, and hinder weight loss. Not having enough vitamin D can make your bones weaker. For this, consider at least to start taking regular multivitamins, and in case of extra deficiencies, take specific supplements that are recommended by your healthcare professional.

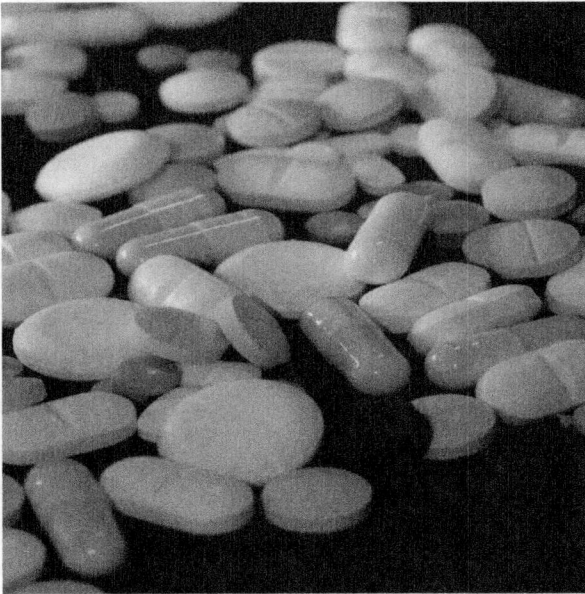

Avoiding Added Sugars

Just like sweetened beverages, we should limit the consumption of sugary foods and desserts like candies, cakes, cookies, ice cream, and sweetened yogurts. Some of the non-obvious foods that often contain added sugars include cereals, dairy-free milk substitutes, condiments like ketchup and other sauces, salad dressings, canned soups, and granola bars. Some of the foods on this list can be surprising and it is unrealistic to expect to completely cut these foods from our diets. A few things that might help are reducing the consumption of such foods, finding alternatives by checking the package labels for "added sugars" tags, and generally, becoming more aware of the foods that are high in sugar content. As we start becoming more cognizant of these things, we will automatically shift towards better eating habits.

Avoiding Convenience Foods

Convenience food can be classified as any of the ready-to-eat foods, fast foods, or overly processed foods that are now commonly available everywhere. You might think that excluding those kinds of foods can make life very challenging, especially for people who have a limited amount of time available to cook fresh food every day. Avoiding processed foods and fast foods will definitely add to your cooking time but with proper meal prep and planning, you can make cooking fresh food every day or every few days easy and enjoyable. While we won't go into much detail about meal prep in this book, there is a lot of material available nowadays that can help you include planning and preparation into your cooking to make it easy and enjoyable.

Including More Home-Cooked Meals

As discussed above, including home-cooked meals in your diet can significantly impact your mind as well as your physical abilities. The degree of freshness of your meals can possibly impact how your body digests it and the level of nutrients it absorbs. Since home-cooked meals are the freshest meals available to us, we should try to incorporate more of them into our diet. Cooking at home gives us more control over the quality of the food that we consume and helps us control the balance of the meal to include all major food groups, limit oil consumption, and other small but important decisions.

Eating More Protein

Ensuring a healthy balance of macronutrients in every meal is important. But as we age, the role of protein in our diet becomes even more important as we need protein to maintain our muscle and bone health. The muscle mass in our body can impact our Resting Metabolic Rate (RMR) which makes sure that we are burning enough calories to maintain a healthy weight, even when resting (Nowson & O'Connell, 2015). Including more protein in your diet as you start an exercise routine can help you build more muscles, which would, in turn, improve your RMR and also protect you from injuries or reduce the impact of injuries and falls.

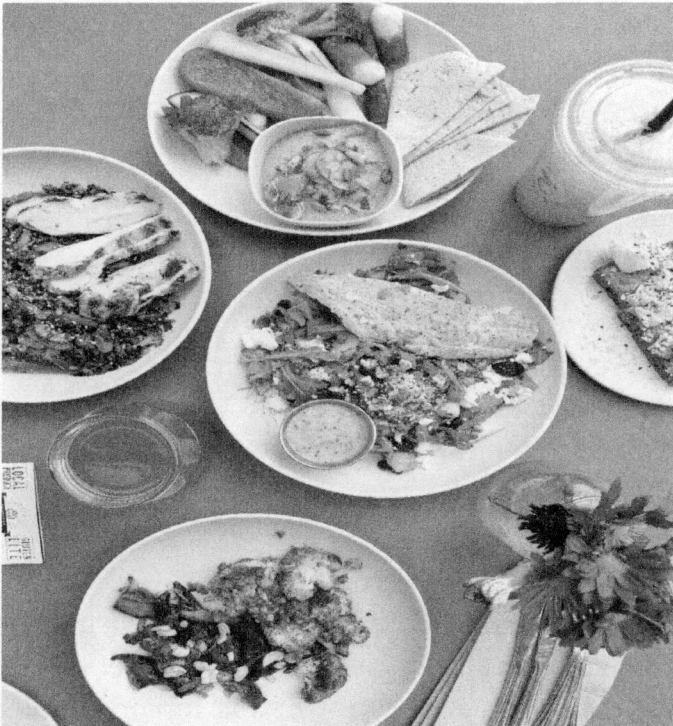

Mindful Eating

A simple way to improve your dietary habits is by eating mindfully, which basically means paying more attention to your food while you are busy eating. One aspect of mindful eating is examining your urge to eat between meals to understand if you are actually hungry or if you just feel like eating for the sake of eating. This can help you improve your eating patterns and may even reduce the quantity of food you eat. It can also help you improve your relationship with food and take an important step toward dealing with other mental issues like emotional eating.

Mindful eating doesn't have specific guidelines, but eating at a leisurely pace, savoring the aroma and flavor of each bite of food, and being aware of your feelings at mealtimes are simple ways to introduce mindful eating to your daily routine.

What Should I Eat?

Now that we have taken a deeper look at some of the habits we can develop to get the best out of our diets to support our chair yoga journey, let's explore some of the foods we should include more of in our diets to gain maximum benefits.

Chronic Inflammation

With age, chronic inflammation, which is when the body is inflamed, typically on the inside, for longer periods of time, becomes a common problem. Chronic inflammation is the body's response to an imbalance, infection, or an untreated chronic condition. Because of the nature of this inflammation, it often goes unnoticed until the condition gets really bad. It is linked to several other chronic diseases like diabetes, heart disease, cancer, arthritis, and bowel diseases like Crohn's disease and ulcerative colitis (Ferrucci & Fabbri, 2018). So, as we age, managing inflammation becomes more important than when we were younger. Nowadays, the condition of having elevated levels of pro-inflammatory markers in the blood is called "inflammaging." As seniors are more susceptible to inflammaging, it also increases the risk of chronic morbidity, disability, frailty, and premature death. So, let's first look at the foods that cause inflammation and then at foods that can break the inflammation cycle.

Inflammatory Foods

Foods With Excess Added Sugars

Foods like bread, crackers, certain salad dressings, and sweets contain added sugars that can cause weight gain and inflammation, and raise bad cholesterol.

Excessive Red Meat or Processed Meats

These types of foods, like bacon, hot dogs, and sausage, are very high in saturated fat, which can increase inflammation in the body.

Excessive Foods Rich in Omega-6s

Our bodies require a healthy balance of omega-6 and omega-3 fatty acids. However, eating too much omega-6, which is found in fatty foods like canola oil, mayonnaise, and peanut oil, can cause a disbalance contributing to chronic inflammation.

Concentrated Refined Carbohydrates

Although these can be part of a healthy diet, refined carbs, like white rice, white bread, and pasta, can break down as simple sugars when eaten and lead to increased inflammation, so they should be eaten in moderation.

Raw or Undercooked Eggs, Meat, and Poultry

Consuming undercooked foods, specifically eggs, poultry, meat, and sushi, can result in food poisoning, which can lead to sepsis and septic shock. Although anyone can develop sepsis (the body's extreme reaction to an infection), the elderly are more susceptible to this.

Grapefruit

If you have been prescribed certain medications for treating high blood pressure, anxiety, or insomnia, you may have been cautioned not to eat grapefruit. The reason is that grapefruit and grapefruit juice can intensify the effects of certain medications, potentially making them dangerous. Check your medication labels to see if it mentions avoiding grapefruit, and if it does, make sure to avoid it!

High-Sodium Foods

Excessive salt in older adults can be a problem, especially those who have hypertension issues. If your meals seem bland with a lack of flavor, consider incorporating different herbs and spices rather than using table salt. It's important to read how much sodium content there is on nutritional labels. According to recommendations from the National Academies of Sciences, Health and Medicine Division (*8 Foods Older Adults Should Avoid Eating*, 2016), seniors over 71 should make sure to have no more than 1.2 grams of sodium per day.

Caffeine

Caffeine not only disrupts sleep patterns for many people, it may also exacerbate anxiety and lead to a rapid or irregular heartbeat. This could be dangerous if you have a heart condition. It is important to note that caffeine is present not only in coffee but in many chocolates, sodas, and teas. Also, make sure to check medications, including painkillers and daytime cough medications, for caffeine content.

Sodas and Sugary Drinks

Sodas and many sports drinks contain large amounts of sugar. Sports drinks especially since their intended effect is to quickly refill the energy and electrolyte deficit caused by playing intense sports. If you have prediabetes, drinking these types of liquids regularly could dangerously raise your blood sugar levels to a diagnosis of diabetes. Excess sugar intake also leads to obesity and other health issues.

"Sugar-Free" Drinks

At first sight, a drink or food product containing artificial sweeteners might seem like a favorable substitute for products high in sugar, but it usually isn't. There is research suggesting artificial sweeteners contribute to weight gain and cause other health problems (*8 Foods Older Adults Should Avoid Eating*, 2016). Although these drinks have relatively lower calories, which is why most people like to drink them, the sugar content will still have negative health implications.

Alcoholic Beverages

Most people may get away with enjoying an occasional alcoholic beverage. However, you will need to avoid it if you have diabetes or take certain types of medications, such as antihistamines, painkillers, or blood pressure medication. Further, according to the Canadian Centre on Substance Use and Addiction (2023), even moderate consumption of 3-6 standard drinks per week can increase your chances of developing various forms of cancer, including breast and colon cancer. Be careful!

Foods With Empty Calories

Even though they might satisfy your cravings, easy and fast foods, such as pizza and pastries lack essential nutrients. What is more, if you only consume fast foods, you may start developing nutrient deficiencies. Seniors have the added challenge of a metabolism that slows down as they become less active with age, making the empty calories from these foods more difficult to get rid of.

Deli Meats

Deli meats, such as bacon, sausage, and ham, are often seen as a delicious source of protein, but they contain a lot of sodium and harmful additives. These processed meats also often contain nitrates, which can increase the risk of colorectal cancer (Smith, 2019).

Sushi

Sushi and any raw fish should also be eaten with caution. Though some sushi dishes include cooked seafood, it is best to enjoy this food in moderation. Additionally, with its raw ingredients, sushi can also be high in sodium, which contributes to high blood pressure and heart disease, another reason for seniors to be cautious before consuming it.

Unpasteurized Dairy and Juice

Due to their rich calcium content, milk and other dairy products are highly recommended for bone health. However, seniors should avoid unpasteurized juice and soft cheeses because they can potentially harbor harmful bacteria, and they should steer clear of unpasteurized milk due to the higher risk of foodborne illness.

Anti-inflammatory Foods

Now that we know which foods cause inflammation, let's look at some common foods that can counter inflammation. Foods that reduce inflammation are the typical, healthy foods that most experts regularly recommend.

Berries

Berries, including acai, blackberries, raspberries, blueberries, and strawberries, are high in antioxidants and are a great option to help target inflammation. You can add these to a meal or have some as a snack.

Avocados

Avocados contain healthy sugar and are an excellent source of healthy fats that help block the pro-inflammatory response in your body. Add avocado or even homemade guacamole to your breakfast for a tasty and nutritious meal.

Grapes

Grapes contain antioxidants, anthocyanins, and resveratrol, which help reduce inflammation.

Cherries

The results of one study showed that eating 45 cherries a day considerably reduced inflammation in patients (Kelley et. al., 2018). You don't have to eat that many cherries every day. Merely including it in your diet can help reduce inflammation.

Mushrooms

Mushrooms are rich in selenium, and bell peppers are rich in B vitamins, phenols, and copper, which offer anti-inflammatory protection. However, it's important not to overcook them, as they will lose these nutrients if overcooked.

Tomatoes

Rich in vitamin C, tomatoes have antioxidants such as potassium, and lycopene which possess anti-inflammatory properties. Adding tomatoes to nearly any dish, from pasta to salads, will give you extra flavor and nutritional benefits.

Kale

Packed with phytonutrients, minerals, and vitamins that fight inflammation, kale is an excellent alternative to romaine in your salad. It's worth a try next time.

Peppers

Chili peppers boast antioxidants and vitamin C, both known for their anti-inflammatory properties. Try it on your next Mexican-inspired dish for a flavorful and healthful boost.

Broccoli

Broccoli is rich in Sulforaphane, an antioxidant with anti-inflammatory properties. You can enjoy this vegetable in various ways: raw, steamed, baked, or sautéed.

Salmon

A rich source of omega-3 fatty acids and DHA, salmon makes for a great choice in having a nutritious lunch or dinner option. Include it with a side of vegetables for a wholesome meal.

Turmeric

Turmeric, a spice renowned for its anti-inflammatory, antimicrobial, and antioxidant properties, can be combined with your culinary creations or even enjoyed in tea.

Dark Chocolate

Dark chocolate contains cocoa, an antioxidant known for its anti-inflammatory properties. Dark chocolate paired with berries makes for a delicious and anti-inflammatory dessert.

Chia seed

Rich in omega-3 fatty acids, chia seeds are known for their anti-inflammatory effects. Add them to your hot cereal or smoothie by incorporating them for a nutritional boost.

Ginger

Ginger contains gingerol, a potent compound known for its anti-inflammatory properties. It also boasts antioxidants that combat free radicals and can treat nausea. Incorporate ginger into your diet by steeping it in hot water to make ginger tea or putting it in fish dishes or soups for added flavor and health benefits.

Carrots

Carrots are plentiful with vitamin A, crucial for regulating the body's inflammatory response and mitigating inflammation. However, excessive consumption of vitamin A over an extended period isn't recommended as it may lead to vitamin toxicity, characterized by symptoms such as bone pain, skin changes, and impaired vision.

Spinach

Spinach is an excellent anti-inflammatory food with many other benefits. Dark leafy greens like spinach are renowned for their high levels of vitamin E compared to lighter-colored counterparts. The vitamin E in spinach acts as an antioxidant that combats free radicals that may contribute to diseases like cancer. Incorporating spinach into your diet is simple. You can even put it in your smoothies for a nutritional boost.

As we look at these different foods and label them as good or bad for our health, it is important to note that none of these foods are inherently good or bad and should not be overused or completely shunned. To maintain a healthy balance, we should reduce the consumption of the food we deem bad and incorporate foods that we deem good. But everything should be in moderation and with consideration to any existing health conditions. When introducing or eliminating any foods from your diet, do it gradually so that your body can acclimatize to the change. Only make major dietary changes at the advice of dieticians or nutritionists along with the guidance of your healthcare professional.

I cannot remember the books I've read any more than the meals I have eaten; even so, they have made me.

— Ralph W. Emerson

Always consider how your diet affects your lifestyle because I'm sure you've heard, you are what you eat, which can interfere with your ability to manage chronic pain or improve mobility if the foods cause inflammation. Also, shedding a few pounds can relieve some pressure on your joints. You can still enjoy food while doing chair yoga, but choose the right foods. Then, you're ready to establish your mind-body connection to ensure your mental health doesn't undo your chair yoga practice.

Food Checklist

Fruits

- Apples
- Avocados
- Bananas
- Berries: blackberries, blueberries, strawberries, raspberries
- Citrus fruits: grapefruit, lemons, limes, oranges
- Grapes
- Kiwis
- Melons
- Pears
- Pomegranates
- Tomatoes

Vegetables

- Asparagus
- Broccoli
- Brussels sprouts
- Cauliflower

- Celery
- Cucumbers
- Garlic
- Ginger
- Green beans
- Kale
- Lettuces

- Mushrooms
- Onions
- Peppers
- Spinach
- Sweet potatoes
- Zucchini

Meats and Proteins

- Eggs (or egg alternatives)
- Hummus
- Lean meats: fish, poultry, turkey
- Low-fat or fat-free cheese and cottage cheese

- Low-fat or fat-free plain Greek or skyr yogurt
- Dairy-alternative milk and yogurts
- Soy: tofu, tempeh

Other foods

- Nuts and seeds: almonds, cashews, walnuts, chia, flax, hemp, sunflower seeds
- Oil and vinegar: apple cider vinegar, avocado oil, olive oil, balsamic vinegar, red or white wine vinegar, rice wine vinegar

- Herbs and spices: basil, cinnamon, cumin, garlic powder, onion powder, oregano, thyme, turmeric, red pepper flakes, etc.

- Whole grain cereal

- Whole grains: oats, quinoa, wild rice

- Dark Chocolate

CHAPTER 4

How the Mind-Body Connection Provides Added Benefits

Mind-Body connection? What has the mind got to do with exercise and chair yoga, you might think? Sure, motivation and discipline are needed, but what else?

Turns out, your mental health and your mind-body connection can absolutely make or break your chair yoga practice. Sadly, one in four seniors suffer from mental health conditions including depression and anxiety. Not improving your mental and cognitive state could unravel the benefits you may otherwise experience from chair yoga. My mother didn't have her chair yoga routine under wraps until she took care of her mind-body connection. Then, the benefits truly showed. Understanding how poor mental health affects your chair yoga benefits will reveal why you must work on your mind-body connection while practicing the sequences.

What Is Mind-Body Connection?

Understanding the Mind-Body Connection

This is the relationship between our thoughts, feelings, attitudes, and our physical health and well-being. This relationship is a complex interconnection where each component influences and relies on the other. In other words, our physical state and how we treat our bodies directly influence our mental health, while our minds directly influence our physical health. This is why what we eat, how much we exercise, and even our posture is important. To understand this better, let's look at the story of a young woman as shared by the University of Minnesota, paraphrased (Hart, 2019, p.1).

Julie appears to have it all – she's well-educated, watches what she eats, she's attractive with a successful career, has a Ph.D., and has a great group of friends. However, there's more to her story. Despite her outward success, Julie grapples with diabetes and anxiety related to her business responsibilities. She often experiences self-directed anger and frustration, occasionally snapping at others over minor mistakes. Even with careful monitoring of her blood sugar levels, Julie finds herself in a coma once or twice a month.

It becomes evident that Julie's anxiety hampers her ability to recognize the signs of low blood sugar despite her otherwise healthy habits. Acting on her doctor's advice, Julie incorporates Mindfulness Based Stress-Reduction (MBSR) classes into her diabetes care regimen. Through these practices, she learns to slow down and tune in to her body's signals.

With improved awareness, Julie becomes better equipped to detect when her blood sugar is dropping, enabling her to take preventative measures and avoid diabetic emergencies. Additionally, managing her anxiety contributes to better diabetes control, possibly by reducing stress hormones. As a result, her anger dissipates, stemming from the stress of her condition.

This story demonstrates how a good mind-body connection can transform your life. When we explore the mind-body connection, one important thing to understand is that the "mind" in this connection does not refer to the brain, but rather our mental state, which includes a combination of our thoughts, feelings, emotions, attitudes, and beliefs. The brain is the physical part of our bodies that allows us to experience this mental state.

Our mental state is not something we are always fully aware of. In some situations, we might have an intense reaction to something without being fully aware of why we are reacting that way. Each mental state has positive or negative effects associated with it. Anxiety, for example, can manifest in the physical body and produce stress hormones.

Historically, the mind-body connection and the role of the mind in your health have always been important. Up until about 300 years ago, most medical systems regarded the mind and body as one entity, treating them holistically. However, during the 17th century, the Western world started viewing these as two distinct entities (Hart, 2019). The body was viewed as something made up of its various physical parts with no connection to the mind. This belief became the foundation of Western medicine and influenced how patient care, surgery, trauma care, and medicines developed.

Although there were great medical advancements, the role of the mind in healing the body was ignored and it also greatly reduced the exploration into humans' emotional and spiritual lives.

During the 20th century, there was a gradual rediscovery of this interconnection. Researchers dug deeper into studying the mind-body relationship, discovering complex links between the two entities through scientific inquiry (Hart, 2019).

Effects of Poor Mental Health on Physical Health

Depression and anxiety are some of the most common mental health issues that the older population faces. Let's take a look at some of the physical effects of these ailments.

Anxiety

When we're stressed out, our body releases two hormones: adrenaline and cortisol. Commonly referred to as stress hormones, they provide a short-term energy surge, known as an adrenaline rush, enabling us to swiftly navigate potentially dangerous situations.

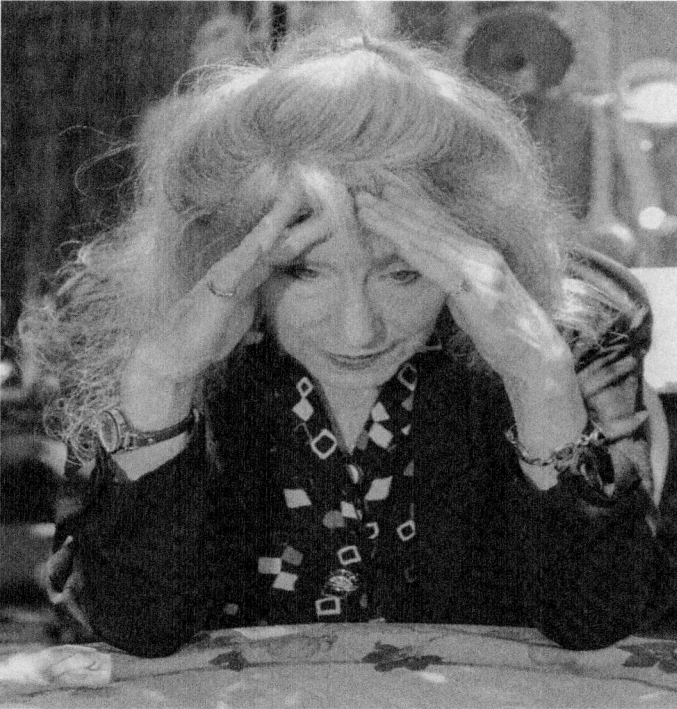

However, you can still feel stressed even if there's no immediate "danger". This prolonged stressed state is what we call anxiety. Releasing stress hormones too frequently can have negative long-term effects on the body, including a weakened immune response, digestive problems, and slower healing times.

While the correlation between stress and health is apparent, for some people, it can be more challenging to grasp that our thoughts and beliefs also play a significant role in influencing our health, too.

Negative thinking patterns like assuming the worst, jumping to conclusions, and self-criticism, to name a few, can make it more difficult to deal with if you're also facing health problems.

Depression

Depression, while primarily a mental disorder, can play a heavy role in appetite and nutrition. Some people cope with stress by emotionally eating, a behavior that can result in serious weight gain and contribute to obesity-related conditions such as type 2 diabetes.

One mental state that is closely related to depression and that can often be a trigger is stress. When we're stressed, hormones are released that elevate heart rate and constrict blood vessels, mimicking a state of emergency. Prolonged exposure can lead to heart disease, as people grappling with depression have an increased risk of cardiovascular conditions.

Having depression can worsen existing health conditions, and cause inflammation, chronic pain, and even cause gastrointestinal problems.

Mental Health and Disease Management in Seniors

Effective management of chronic diseases requires a change to your lifestyle, including eating healthier, exercising regularly, and better sleeping habits. Yet, our capacity to make these changes is influenced by our attitudes, actions, and behaviors, which are ultimately governed by our minds. Mindset is everything!

Wellness is as much of a mental battle as it is physical. According to a 2011 survey by the APA, about 27% of Americans said that the reason they were not making the lifestyle changes they knew they had to make was a lack of willpower. Even if we have the desire to change, our mind is still the determining factor. Our thought patterns, worries, fears, and anxieties can either guide us toward wellness or lead us astray from it.

A drop in mental health, increase in stress and anxiety as well as depression can be linked to an increased likelihood of chronic diseases, ulcers, and cancers. The detrimental effects of mental health often manifest in physical health as well.

How can a Mind-Body Connection Help with Chair Yoga?

A sound mind-body connection can help create a healthy mental environment to take the most advantage possible of the yoga practices we learn. It is crucial to address this since mental and neurological disorders in older adults account for 6.6% of the total disabilities in this age bracket. About 15% of individuals aged 60 and over suffer from a mental disorder (Pan American Health Organization, n.d.). So, while it will help with your yoga practice, addressing your mental health will also help you improve your quality of life in general.

One easy and extremely natural way to improve your mental health is through social interactions. The impact of social interaction can have profound effects on your health and lifespan. In fact, evidence suggests strong social interactions may be just as important as physical activity and a nutritious diet (Harvard Health Publishing, 2021). Strong social interactions can play a critical role in protecting your memory and cognitive function in several ways as you age.

- Regular social interactions can help you keep up your cognitive functions

- It can help fight off depression, which often goes hand in hand with loneliness and can be connected to faster cognitive decline.

- A robust network of supportive people who care for you can help reduce your stress levels.

- It keeps you engaged in important mental processes such as memory and attention, which can increase awareness.

- Regular engagement aids in reinforcing neural networks, thereby slowing down typical age-related declines.

- It may also contribute to strengthening cognitive reserve, which can delay the onset of dementia.

While this can be one easy way to improve your mental health, you still need to strengthen your mind-body connection not just to improve your mental health but also to understand your body more, listen to its cues, and take better care of it.

The mind-body connection is also used as a basis for some mental health therapies that include practices such as yoga, tai chi, and some types of dance. These therapies have a strong focus on how the body affects the mind as well as how the mind affects the body. Other common mind-body therapies include:

- cognitive-behavioral therapy

- meditation

- creative arts therapies (art, music, or dance)

- relaxation

- hypnosis

- guided imagery

Among these, yoga, meditation, and mindfulness are some of the more intuitive and impactful exercises. While all are extremely effective strategies, these three can often be the easiest to grasp and incorporate into our lives.

Mindfulness-based treatments that help patients to focus on the present can have a positive impact on their health and well-being. These treatment therapies help to reduce anxiety and depression, and there's also evidence that mindfulness can lower blood pressure and improve sleep (National Institutes of Health, 2021). It may even help people deal with pain better. "For many chronic illnesses, mindfulness meditation seems to improve quality of life and reduce mental health symptoms," says Dr. Zev Schuman-Olivier of Harvard University (National Institutes of Health, 2021). In recent years, mindfulness and meditation have also become part of behavioral therapies used to treat depression and anxiety.

Improving Mind-Body Connection Through Mindfulness

Now that we know what the mind-body connection is and its benefits to our yoga practice as well as in life, let's take a closer look at mind-body therapies to improve our mindfulness and the mind-body connection.

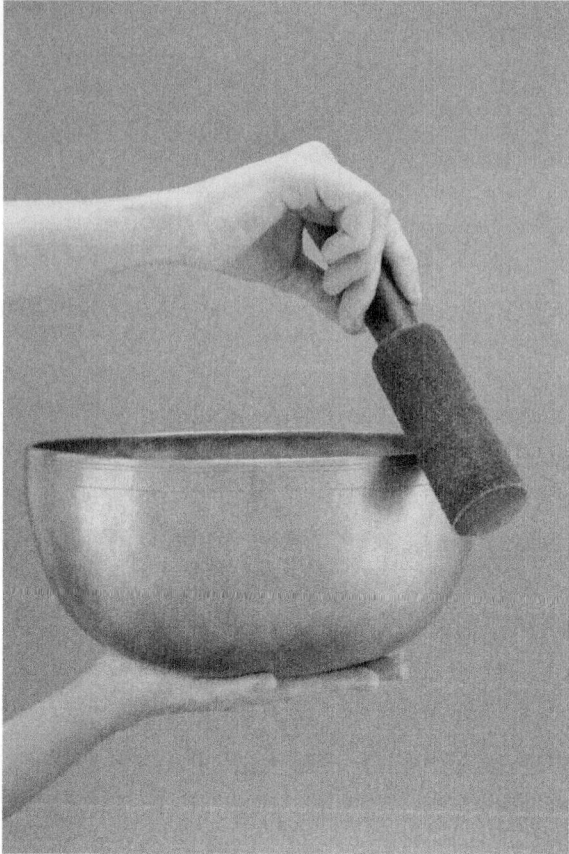

Some people get confused by the difference between meditation and mindfulness. As the name might indicate, it is a type of awareness. When you are mindful, or aware, of what is happening in your body as you perform certain actions or when you are in a certain emotional state, that awareness is called mindfulness. Being mindful means, being aware of how you feel and what sensations you are experiencing in your body in the moment, without judging it or trying to figure out what these feelings mean. Numerous tools are available to practice mindfulness, including breathing methods, guided imagery, and other methods aimed at relaxing the body and mind. So, meditation is a way of practicing mindfulness as through the meditation process, you focus on your breath and what is going on in your body.

Practicing mindfulness can help you deal with all the daily distractions and stressors, such as planning your schedule, problem-solving, and managing crises. It can also assist in combating negative thoughts that drain your mind. Not dealing with these stressors makes you more prone to stress, anxiety, and depression.

Mindfulness can often be deceptively easy to practice. All you need to do is keep your focus and pay attention. Here are some very easy and common ways you can practice mindfulness are described next. You can do them at any point in the day, even during the chair yoga practice.

- **Pay attention.** When you have a busy lifestyle, it can be tricky to get your mind to slow down. Focusing on the world around you through your senses. Through touch, sound, sight, smell, and taste, you can be more present and pay attention. For example, when you eat, take the time to smell, taste, and truly enjoy it.

- **Live in the moment.** Be intentional in the way you interact with the world. Try finding joy in simple pleasures. Nowadays, people have started looking for "glimmers" that make you happy and are the opposite of triggers. They are supposed to remind you to be present and enjoy the little things.

- **Accepting yourself.** Always treat yourself with the same kindness and compassion you would treat a good friend.

Focus on your breathing. When negative thoughts occur, sit down, take a deep breath, and gently close your eyes. Direct your focus on your breath as you inhale and exhale. Sitting and breathing for even just a moment can help. Here is one simple breathing technique that you can practice whenever you need to center yourself.

o Start by finding a comfortable position; it could be seated, lying down, or standing up.

o Close your eyes and pay attention to your breathing as you inhale and exhale.

o Try breathing in 5-second cycles; inhale for 5 seconds, hold for 5, exhale for 5 seconds, then repeat the process.

o As you breathe in and out, pay attention to the sensations in your body. If you find your thoughts drifting, gently redirect your attention back to your breath.

o Feel free to continue this exercise for as long as it feels comfortable for you. Try starting with five minutes and adjust from there.

When you try mindfulness, it can be daunting. Fortunately, there are many apps and resources available to guide both beginners and advanced practitioners of mindfulness.

Mindfulness Podcasts

You can try listening to any of the free mindfulness podcasts that can help you with meditation and breathing techniques. Some of the most popular podcasts are:

- *The Meditation Podcast.* Narrated by Jesse and Jeane Stern, this podcast offers easy meditations to help listeners deal with mental health issues like stress and depression. They also use audio tones that help with relaxation.

- *Guided Meditations by Tara Brach.* Tara Brach is the founder of Insight Meditation Community of Washington, DC, which is one of the largest meditation centers in the United States. In this podcast, she combines her background in psychotherapy with training in Buddhist techniques to create content for listeners looking to balance out their mental states.

- *The Daily Meditation Podcast.* Hosted by Mary Meckley, whose straightforward and genuine approach, makes it feel like you're listening to a friend. There are weekly themes, so there's always something fresh to listen to.

Mindfulness Mobile Phone Apps

You can try all the different mobile phone apps available nowadays for mindfulness practices. They are easy to use and provide you with bite-sized information for easy implementation in your daily life. Some of the most popular apps are:

- *Headspace*. This is a mindfulness app that focuses on guiding you through meditation. It's a good choice for beginners who want to learn more about meditation and discover how to practice it. The app offers unlimited meditation sessions, so you can try it out and see if it works for you.

- *Buddhify*. This is an online meditation app that can help you find a quiet space in your daily life. The app offers several guided meditations on different topics and lengths, so you can pick what works best for you. What is different about this app is you can do this based on what you are feeling at the moment to relieve it; it can be customized according to your needs.

- *Breathe+*. This app helps you visualize your breathing beautifully and simply. Whether you want to relax daily, meditate, or train your breathing, this app has the resources for you.

- *Calm*. This is an excellent meditation app that features guided meditations and sleep stories. It has been designed specifically with seniors in mind, so it's easy to use and understand. It also features calming music that will help you feel better about yourself.

As we look at the various ways to introduce mindfulness into our lives, we may wonder how often one needs to practice this. The answer is, it depends on what kind of mindfulness exercise you plan to do.

Mindfulness exercises are so easy and unobtrusive that you can practice them anywhere and anytime. A great way to engage all your senses is to practice them outdoors or in nature. If you prefer something more structured, choose a specific team each day and find a designated spot where you can practice without being interrupted. You can even combine your chair yoga and mindfulness practices and make them part of your morning or daily routine.

Instead of focusing on the number of hours or minutes you need to put in per day, focus on the consistency of your practice. Start small with an aim to practice mindfulness every day for a week, reflect on your experience at the end of the week, and then commit yourself to do it again the next week. Over time, you may discover that mindfulness becomes effortless. Think of it as a commitment to nurturing yourself to bring out the best version of yourself.

Emotional Awareness

Mindfulness techniques can help you when you are feeling overwhelmed or emotional. When you commit to practicing mindfulness whenever you feel emotional or stressed, you can control the hormones that could undo chair yoga benefits. But this is easier said than done. To control and manage your emotions in stressful situations, you need to become aware of your emotions. For this, you need to practice emotional awareness when you are not in a highly emotional state so that you can learn to recognize your emotions better. There is a simple emotional awareness meditation that you can follow for this developed by the Mindfulness Meditation Institute (n.d.). The main objective is to train yourself with the ability to observe your emotions. Through regular practice, this form of meditation will empower you to gain more control over your emotions and develop greater inner strength.

To practice emotional awareness meditation, make sure you are completely relaxed and in a place where you won't be disturbed for some time. Focus on your breathing and count each breath inhalation and exhalation — silently in your mind. When you get to five, just start over again. Keep your focus on the air passing through the tip of your nose. Whenever your mind starts wandering, immediately focus on your breath instead.

Once you are focused, pose this question to yourself, "What am I feeling?" Are you happy, sad, lonely, angry, restless, bored, or some other emotion? Do not put any judgment towards the emotion, just feel the feeling. Some emotions that arise from your subconscious mind may be subtle and harder to identify. They tend to manifest themselves without seemingly any rhyme or reason and affect your entire mindset.

Once you have mastered the basics of emotional awareness meditations, there are additional steps in the practice you can explore, but for now, direct your attention on identifying the emotions within you. If you're ready, you can explore those emotions deeper. Consider the thoughts behind them and try to look at the situations differently, that is, from a broader perspective.

Guided Imagery

Another method of practicing mindfulness and meditation to improve your mind-body connection is through guided imagery-based meditations. These meditations are available on a variety of apps and podcasts that take you through a guided meditation using imagery to help bring you peace and calm yourself as well as seek guidance. It is quite easy to find these on YouTube just by searching "guided meditation." You can also look up classes or meditation groups in your area.

Music Therapy

While it may sound fancy, it really is one of the easiest ways of bringing more mindfulness into your life. Music holds great potential as a tool for relaxation and meditation. Choosing a song you find restful is a great way to begin. Ensure that the music is not too loud or fast or something that may cause you agitation. Once the song is playing, focus entirely on the music. Keep your eyes open or closed, but keep your gaze soft and avoid focusing on anything around you. Find a comfortable spot and spend a few minutes immersing yourself in your song choice. The act of listening to a simple song has the ability to alter your mindset for the rest of the day.

Chair Yoga and Mindfulness

You may notice that all the mindfulness practices we have discussed are things you can or should do outside of your chair yoga practice. And if you don't have that much extra time on your hands, there are ways you can combine your daily mindfulness practice and chair yoga practices. Let's look at some of the things you can do to make your chair yoga practice more mindful.

Body Scans

You can do this practice before your chair yoga practice to bring yourself to the present and even help you set intentions for your session. Lie on your back with your legs extended, or sit comfortably with arms at your sides, or on your lap, palms facing up. Focus your attention deliberately on each part of your body, in sequence, from toe to head or head to toe. As you focus on each part of the body, consciously relax it, bringing your awareness to any sensations, emotions, or thoughts associated with that part of your body.

Walking meditation

This can also be done right before your chair yoga session, it will also help you release stiffness from your body and as part of the warmup. Find a quiet place where you have at least 10 to 20 feet of open space, and begin to walk slowly. You can do this outside as well but make sure that you are undisturbed and your focus will not be diverted. Pay attention to the experience of walking, and be aware of all the sensations you are feeling. Any sensation like standing, moving, or the subtle adjustments that keep your balance. When you reach the end of your path, pivot and continue walking, maintaining awareness of your sensations.

Mindful Stretching

Yoga and meditation have a richly connected past. During your yoga practice, be attentive to the sensations of your body as you navigate different poses and stretches. Focusing on and moving your body this way is both a mindfulness practice and a workout simultaneously. By just remaining mindful of every stretch during your chair yoga sequences, and noticing how your body's physical sensations change, you can enhance your chair yoga practice to be a mindfulness practice as well.

A Simple Meditation

Next, let's take a look at a simple meditation that you can do before bed or anytime you wish to. This simple practice can bring a much-needed balance into your life and make you more in tune with your body.

1. Sitting in an upright position or lying down on your back, find a comfortable position you can sustain for a few minutes.

2. As you gently bring your awareness to your breath, release any tension present in your body.

3. You only need to observe your breath, do not change anything.

4. Observe the movements and sensations in your body with each inhalation and exhalation.

5. As the air passes through your nose and throat to your lungs, feel the expansion of the chest and belly. Follow the breath in a similar way as you exhale.

6. Continue doing this for a few minutes.

If you are distressed by anything external, the pain is not due to the thing itself, but to your estimate of it; and this you have the power to revoke at any moment.

—Marcus Aurelius

Controlling your mind helps you manage your body. You control your thoughts and feelings and can slow down any decline with simple practices. Then, you're well-prepared to take the next step, which is all about breathing and circulation, two more physical aspects related to chair yoga. Proper breathing techniques and light cardio can help you improve your physical benefits from chair yoga. Let's discover how in the next strategy.

CHAPTER 5

Breathe Deeper and Welcome Light Cardio to Chair Yoga

B efore we get into the chair yoga sequences, there is one more step to discuss that has to do with preparing your body and mind. This involves learning two more practices to ensure good heart health, mental sharpness, and physical well-being. These practices are breathwork and light cardio. When you can understand and incorporate these two practices, you will be fully equipped to start chair yoga. It will go a long way toward helping you improve your independence and wellness through chair yoga.

Cardio is an almost overused term in the health and fitness industry. Whether you love it or hate it, even chair yoga practitioners will agree, you can't ignore it. You might have thought your practices have more to do with sitting, so why do we need cardio? We need cardio because improving your heart health and lung capacity is an important part of chair yoga.

Along with cardio, breathwork can also support heart and lung health, with the ultimate purpose of improving the body's endurance. Breathwork or Yogic breathing refers to breathing techniques that match yoga poses and transitions for optimum yoga practice, but you can do them without the asanas (yoga poses) as well to improve circulation and reap other physical and mental benefits. Yoga is nothing without knowing how to breathe properly, so discovering breathing techniques can enhance your practice. The mind-body connection also means your body affects your mind and, in this case, your brain's health. These two methods can help resolve the threat to your mental health, which can also undo your physical benefits from chair yoga.

Understanding the Importance of Breathwork and Cardio

What Is Cardiovascular Exercise or Cardio?

We all know how the lungs and heart work together to provide us oxygen and energy, but let's take a refresher to understand how it works so that we can grasp more intuitively how it all comes together and why cardio can be so important. Your lungs are a major part of your body's respiratory system. On each inhale, your lungs fill with oxygen, and on each exhale you release carbon dioxide. When you fill your lungs with oxygen, it is released into your bloodstream and pumped through the rest of your body via your arteries.

Through this process, the carbon dioxide in your blood gets filtered through your lungs and replaced with oxygen, which gives you that breath of fresh air.

When you exercise, your body needs more oxygen, and your breathing and heart rate increase, especially when you are running or doing cardiovascular exercise — or cardio. The heightened rate helps your body meet the demands of your exercise.

By the age of 20-25, our lungs mature and after the age of about 35, lung function starts to decline slowly, making breathing slightly more difficult. As you age, your lungs and respiratory system undergo changes. The alveolar dead space in your lungs increases, which affects the amount of oxygen in your arteries without impairing the process of removal of carbon dioxide. The airway receptors also undergo functional changes and may become less sensitive to the medicines that would have worked well when you were younger. The diaphragm muscles may get weaker over time and lung tissue responsible for keeping your airways open can lose elasticity, shrinking your airways. Also, changes in your rib cage bones may occur, reducing the capacity of your lungs to expand. If there are any sudden difficulties in breathing or shortness of breath, talk to your health professional right away, since it might not just be a normal part of aging but an indication of something more serious.

What Is Breathwork?

Breathwork has been an important part of yoga from the start. Not only does it guide your practice, but it also helps you to nourish your body as you breathe in and release stress and toxins as you breathe out.

When you feel stressed, you start taking fast, shallow breaths, which limits the oxygen entering your bloodstream. Your brain perceives this as a sign that there is a threat and puts your body on high alert. In extremely stressful situations, your body then goes into fight-or-flight mode, even if there is no physical threat. Breathwork helps to counteract this; by taking slow, deep, purposeful breaths, you tell your brain that everything is fine and that it can tell your body to relax. Your fight-or-flight response decreases, and your body returns to its normal state. Changing how you breathe can alter your entire body chemistry and your mental state.

How Can Cardio and Breathwork Help?

Breathwork can help to alkalize your blood pH (potential of hydrogen), reduce inflammation, and elevate your mood. It may also have a positive impact on your brain and nervous system. As we discussed before, merely changing how you breathe can change your bodily reactions as well as your mental state. Additional benefits of breathwork are:

- more balanced blood pressure
- better deep sleep
- a reduction of PTSD and feelings of trauma
- an improved respiratory function
- a better immune system
- a release of stress hormones from your body

- reduced feelings of anxiety and depression

- enhanced mental focus

- a reduction in addictive behaviors

- allowing your emotional scars to heal

- a more positive outlook on life

As we look at enjoying all these benefits, it is important to remember that overdoing breathwork can easily escalate it into hyperventilation, which could potentially hurt you. So, always be careful when practicing breathwork.

Light cardio in conjunction with breathwork can even aid in improving lung function. So we can even look at cardio as another form of breathwork. Breathwork can also be extremely helpful when doing cardio or aerobic exercises like running. When you regulate your breath and breathing properly during exercise, you can increase your stamina and get better long-term results. This also means you will be less out of breath.

Cardio and Breathwork Practices to Aid in Chair Yoga

Engaging in breathwork and light chair cardio is essential in your senior years, especially as an active part of your chair yoga routine. Let's explore what you need to ensure your breathwork and cardio support your chair yoga sequences. In all the practices we share, yogic breathing is included as part of the exercise, which means you can do one practice to ensure that both breathwork and cardiovascular exercise are taken care of.

But First, How Much Cardio Do You Need?

According to the Centers for Disease Control and Prevention (2019), adults aged 65 and older require:

- At least **150 minutes a week** (for example, 30 minutes a day, 5 days a week) of moderate-intensity physical activity such as brisk walking, or alternatively, 75 minutes a week of vigorous-intensity activities such as hiking, jogging, or running.

- At least **2 days a week** in muscle-strengthening activities.

- Activities to **improve balance**, such as practicing standing on one foot.

Adults with limited mobility can focus on light cardio activities like moving around the home, walking at a slow pace, cleaning and dusting, vacuuming, making the bed, and standing up. But if you feel up for more intensity than this but not quite to the level of many youngsters, you can consider some of the medium-impact exercises we discuss next. However, as you consider different ways of doing cardio, always remember to prioritize your safety and to only engage in cardio exercises that fit your abilities and are low-impact enough to keep you safe from injuries, especially if you're practicing anything in a standing position or out of a chair.

There are some general guidelines to remember when starting any exercise routine at an advanced age. Always make sure to engage in exercises for your fitness level, and then you can gradually increase your routine from there. Over-exercising can cause injury and may also demotivate you enough to quit. So rather choose a slow and steady pace to ensure your progress. To reduce your risk of injury:

- Always warm up before and cool down after your exercise routine to protect your body from injury.

- Start with low-intensity exercises, that slowly activate your muscles.

- Make sure to choose a safe and secure space when exercising outdoors.

- Keep your body hydrated before, during, and after your workout session, even if you don't feel thirsty.

- Wear appropriate clothes and shoes for your activity.

- If you have any health conditions, it's important to discuss your exercise routines with your healthcare provider.

Now let's look at some low to medium-intensity aerobic exercises next.

Water Aerobics

Water aerobics has become an extremely popular form of exercise, especially for seniors, since the light, natural resistance of the water puts less stress on the joints. For those with arthritis and other forms of joint pain, it is the perfect type of exercise. Water aerobics exercises are a great alternative to strength training and improve your strength, flexibility, and balance with minimal stress on your body. Some popular water aerobic exercises include water walking (low-impact exercise performed in water) or jogging, deep water bicycles, flutter kicks, leg lifts, standing water push-ups, and arm curls.

Pilates

Pilates is a well-known form of exercise that has been around for a century. This low-impact exercise helps build strength while focusing on breathing, body alignment, and core development. It is particularly popular among seniors since practices often involve a combination of accessories including mats, pilates balls, and other inflated accessories for extra support. Pilates also helps older adults to improve balance, develop core strength, and increase flexibility. Pilates exercises suitable for older adults include leg lifts, side circles, arm dips, step-ups, and various plank pose variations, among others.

Tai Chi

Tai chi originated in ancient China, where it started as a martial arts form. As a mind-body exercise, it incorporates slow and gentle movements that are very well-suited for older adults, including those managing chronic conditions. It provides benefits such as flexibility, muscle strengthening, and endurance training. Tai Chi offers seniors with existing impairments, a safe way to improve their health and can be particularly effective as part of strength training in physiotherapy or post-injury rehabilitation. It is also effective for seniors who want to improve their mobility and prevent falling. A review published in the journal PLoS One (Public Library of Science, 2015) found that regular tai chi practice improved cardiovascular health, especially heart and lung health, even in healthy adults.

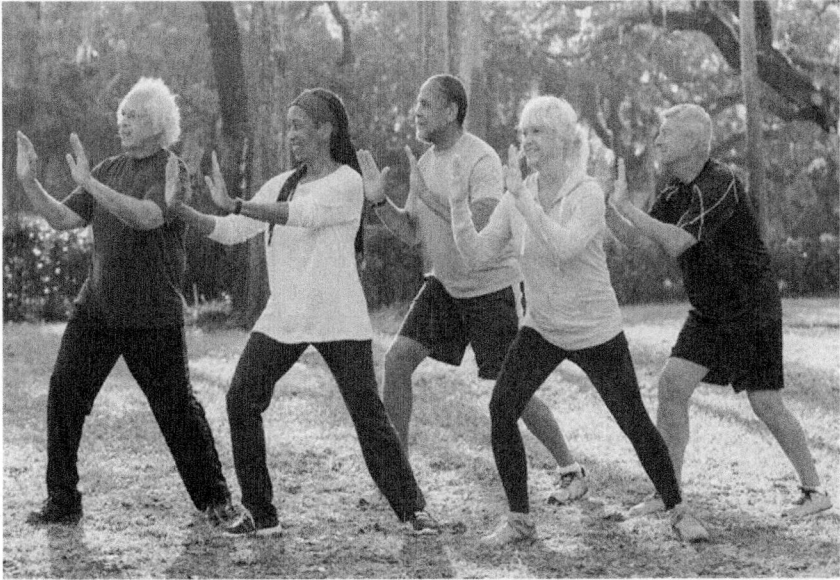

Walking

Walking is probably the most accessible and low-impact form of exercise. For some seniors, walking can also be a significant challenge, so distance and step goals can differ from person to person. Healthcare practitioners advise a daily step count of 10,000 steps to the general public but those with difficulty walking or joint pain can set a smaller number as a goal. According to a study published in PLoS One (Zheng et al., 2015), it found that walking 10,000 steps lowered the ten-year outlook for mortality by 46%. Walking not only promotes a healthy lifestyle while strengthening muscles, it also lowers your risk of heart disease, stroke, diabetes, and colon cancer. Although sometimes walking can also be monotonous. To keep yourself motivated you can:

- find a moderate trail through a park.

- find a walk-friendly race to train for.

- walk the perimeter of a familiar building.

- find an audiobook or a playlist for stimulation during your walk.

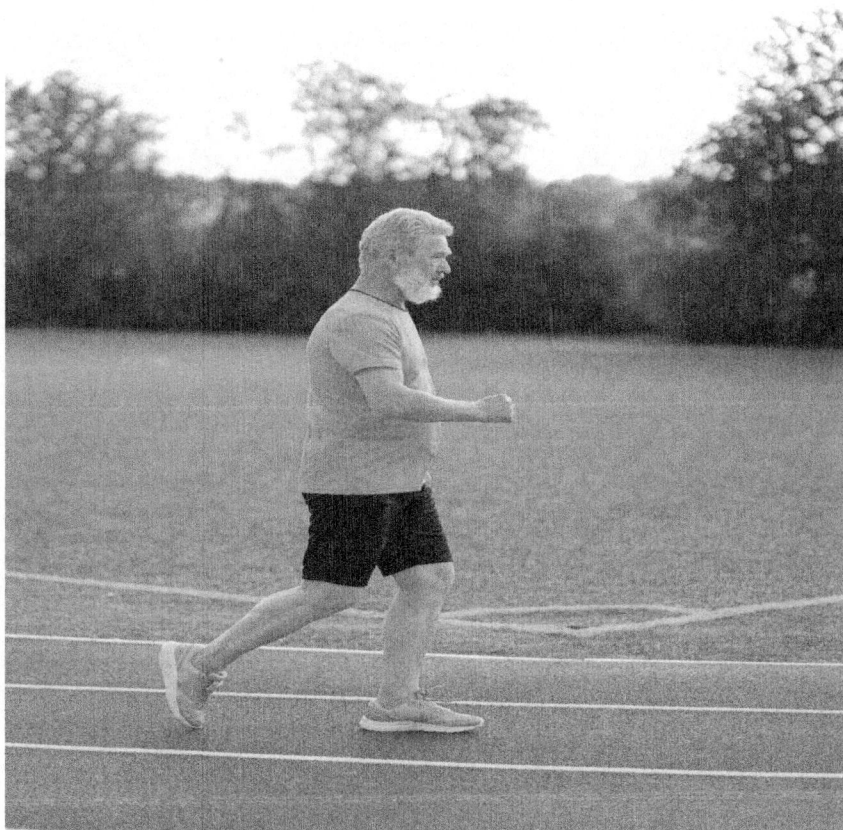

Standing Cardio

We can do cardio exercises just standing (no jumping) and even take the support of the chair for balance and stability. Some of the simpler exercises which you can do are discussed below.

MARCHING

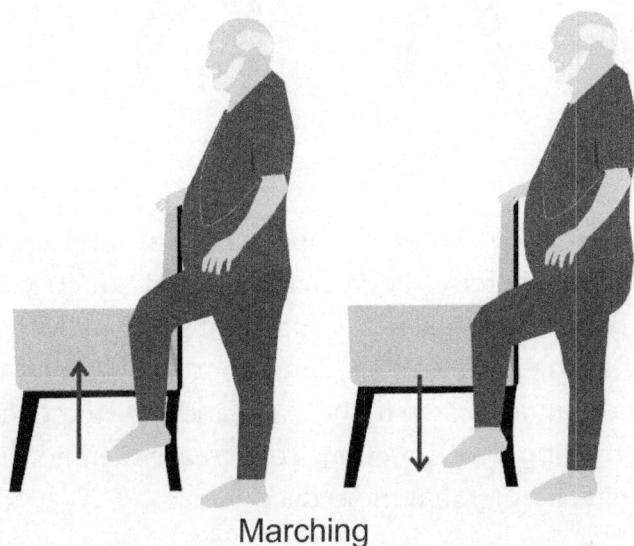

Marching

This straightforward exercise is something anyone can do and is a great way to warm up. Start by placing your hands on your hips while standing, then raise your knee to waist level, lower, and repeat with the opposite leg. Continue this sequence for a minute or even longer to get your heart pumping.

SIDE STEP

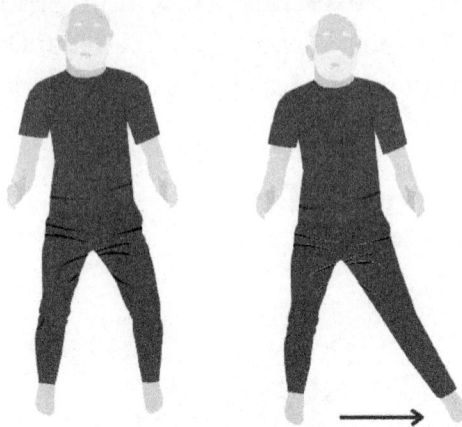

Side Step

Ensure you have sufficient open space around you before you start this exercise. Begin with a slight squat, your legs slightly bent. Next, extend your right leg out to the side, shuffling to the right and bringing your left leg over to meet it. Then take another step to the right, and repeat the sequence going in the opposite direction. To increase the intensity, you can move faster or squat more deeply.

TOE TAPS

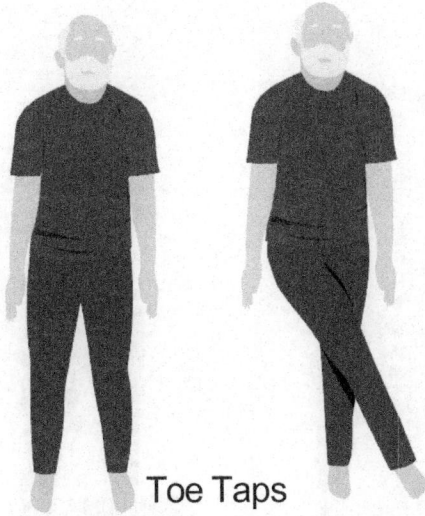

Toe Taps

Begin by standing upright with your feet positioned shoulder-width apart. Next, move your right foot forward, crossing it over to the other side of your opposite leg, and lightly tap the floor with your toe. Then return to your starting position and repeat with the other leg.

HEEL TAPS

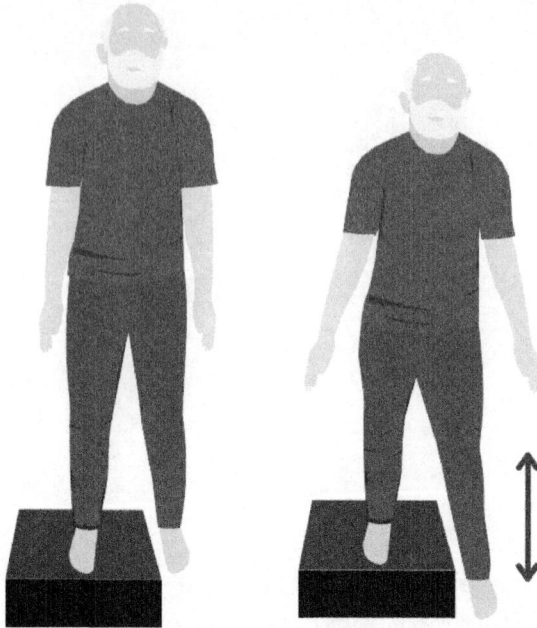

Heel Taps

Here's another exercise you can do using a step. Instead of facing the step directly, position yourself with your right side facing it, leaving one foot on the step and the other hanging off the side. Begin by bending your right leg until the heel of your left foot touches the ground, then return to the starting position. Repeat this process for the opposite leg by facing the opposite direction and performing the same movement.

KNEE RAISES

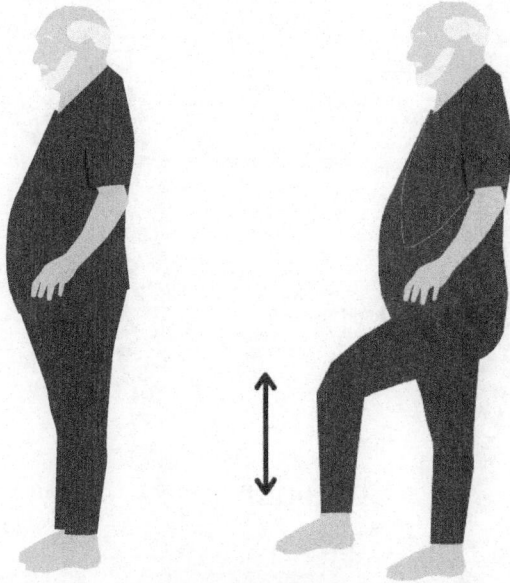

Knee Raises

This is a milder version of marches you can do to ease yourself into a cardio workout. Raise your knee so that it is at a 45-degree angle from the floor. As you progress in the practice you can try raising your leg to waist height, but begin with the smaller raise. Hold for 2-3 seconds, and then lower it to the starting position. Do ten reps for each leg.

SHOULDER RAISES

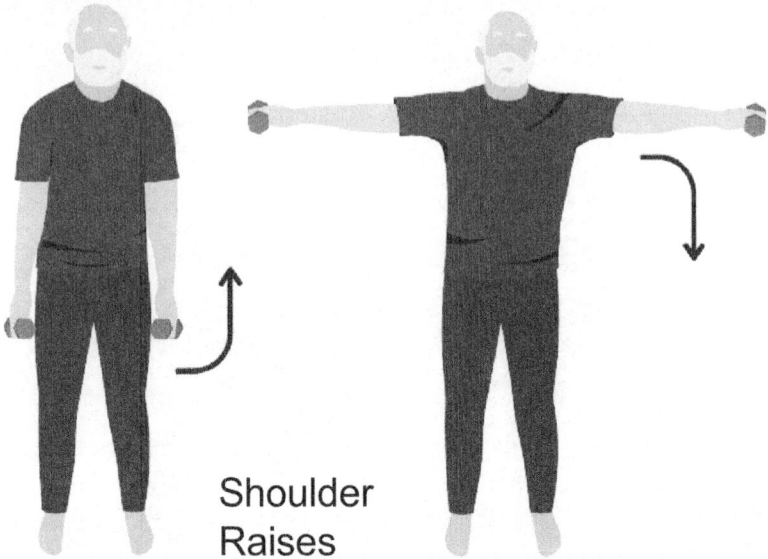

Shoulder
Raises

This exercise can be done with or without hand weights, allowing for an additional challenge or a more relaxed workout. Begin with your arms at your sides while standing tall. Then, simply extend your arms outwards to each side. Then, lower them back to the starting position and begin the process again.

ARM CIRCLES

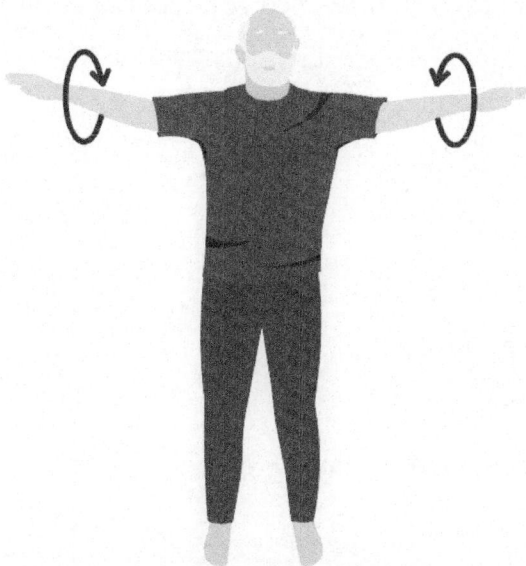

Arm Circles

Holding your arms out to the sides, begin drawing small concentric circles with your hands. Start by moving slowly at first, rotating your arms in small circles, then gradually widening the width for a full shoulder workout. Make sure you don't move too quickly to avoid injury. You can either do all of these cardio exercises as a routine or combine only the ones that suit you.

If You Want to Do More High-Intensity Cardio

Everything we have discussed so far is light to medium-intensity exercises that will help you break a sweat without the risk of injuries. As you progress in your routine, you might want to up the intensity of the exercises. As always, consult your physician before including any risky exercises in your routine. But some of the common high-intensity exercises you can include once you feel ready, are:

- running

- swimming

- tennis

- aerobics

- hiking

- cycling

- various forms of dance

- martial arts

Practice Time!

Next, let's look at some specific breathwork and cardio routines and techniques that we can include in our practices.

DEEP ABDOMINAL BREATHING

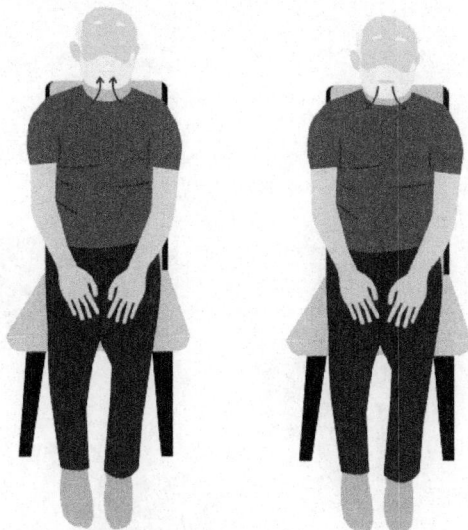

Deep Abdominal Breathing

This technique uses long, deep breathing that helps your body to relax.

1. As you breathe in, visualize your lungs filling up with air, as you expand your belly and chest with each breath.

2. When you exhale, relax your chest, and pull back your navel in towards your spine.

4-7-8 BREATH

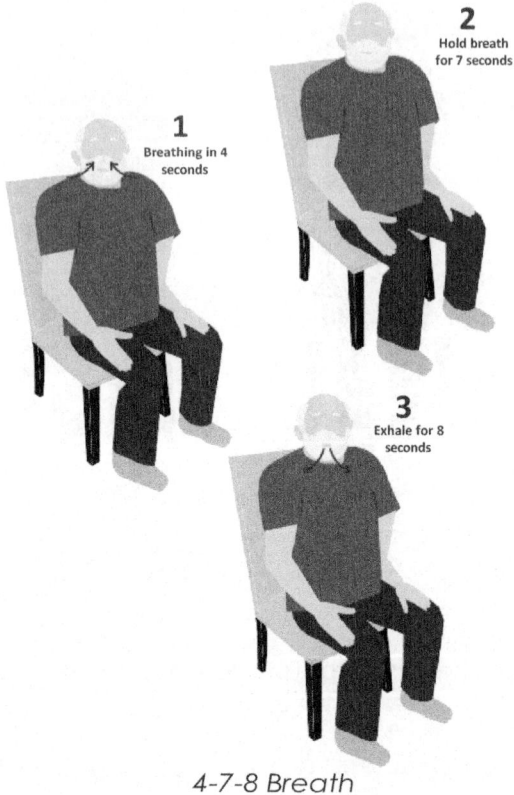

4-7-8 Breath

This technique helps to quiet and focus your mind.

1. Count your breath as you breathe in and out.

2. Count four breaths as you breathe in.

3. Hold your breath for seven counts.

4. Exhale for eight counts.

The longer exhalation in this technique is to ensure that your lungs get completely emptied out.

ALTERNATE NOSTRIL BREATHING

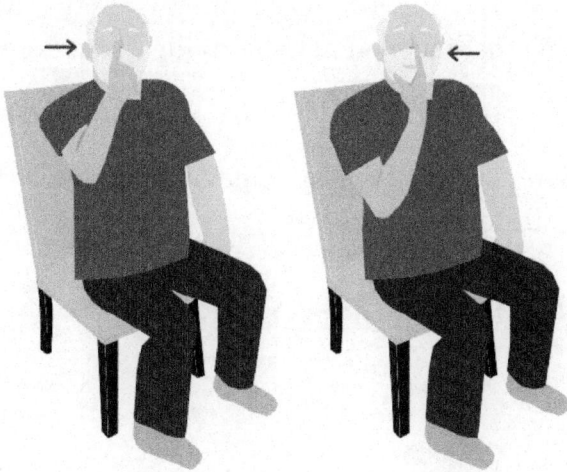

Alternate Nostril Breathing

This breathing technique helps encourage balance in your mind and body.

1. Place your right thumb on your right nostril and apply light pressure.

2. Inhale using only your left nostril and hold your breath as you switch sides.

3. Release your right thumb and, take your right index finger and apply pressure to the left nostril as you breathe out through the right nostril.

4. Pause, take another deep breath in, and then alternate again.

BREATH OF FIRE

This is a more advanced technique that may take a little practice. Once achieved, it helps provide a sense of steadiness.

1. When you inhale, relax your abdominal muscles.

2. When you breathe out, engage your core to help push the air out of your body.

CHINESE OR TAI CHI BREATHING

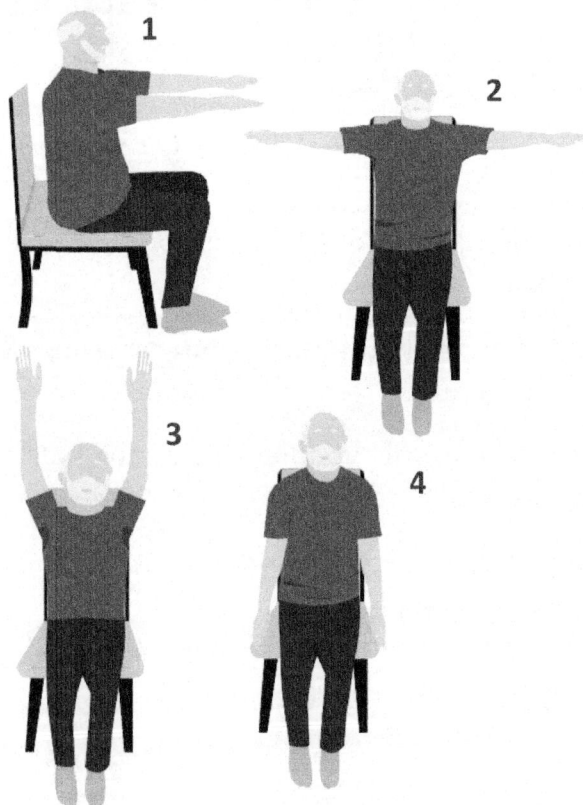

Chinese or Tai Chi Breathing

This comes from the Chinese practice of Tai Chi Chuan.

1. Take three short breaths in.

2. Raise your arms shoulder height in front of you on the first breath.

3. Pull your arms to shoulder height at your sides on your second breath.

4. Raise them above your head on the last breath.

5. Then slowly exhale and lower your arms back down to your sides.

6. Try 10-12 repetitions. **If you get light-headed, stop the exercise.**

BUTEYKO BREATHING

This exercise is particularly helpful for people with breathing problems like asthma. During an asthma attack or stressful situation, it can help slow down the cycle of rapid, gasping breaths.

1. Start by finding a comfortable position in a quiet place.

2. Instead of taking a deep breath, concentrate on taking slow shallow breaths through your nose.

COMPLETE BREATHING

Also called three-part breath, this technique involves engaging the lower ribcage, diaphragm, and upper chest to attain a deep and thorough breath. It covers both belly breathing and chest breathing.

1. Sit up straight and exhale.

2. Start breathing in and relax your stomach muscles.

3. Feel your belly expand as your lungs fill with air.

4. Keep breathing in until you feel your chest expand with a deep breath.

5. Hold your breath briefly and exhale slowly.

6. Pull your belly in to feel the last bit of air leaving your lungs.

7. Close your eyes, relax, and focus on breathing like this for five minutes every day.

DIAPHRAGMATIC BREATHING

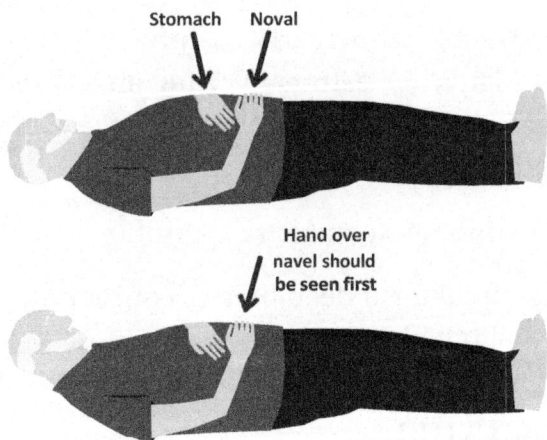

Diaphragmatic Breathing

This promotes relaxation and strengthens the diaphragm muscles.

1. The best position to practice this exercise is to lie down on your back.

2. Place one hand over your navel and your other hand above it on your stomach.

3. Now concentrate on breathing from your diaphragm.

4. If you can see your hand over your navel rising before the hand above it, you are doing this exercise right.

5. Relax and keep breathing for five minutes.

Cardio on a Chair

Next, we look at a sequence of exercises that can be done within 5-10 minutes for a quick cardio exercise. All exercises should be done with smooth movements. Take your time through them, avoiding any jerked movements. Take appropriate breaks between the exercises, but ensure that it is such that your heartbeat picks up.

HIP MARCHING

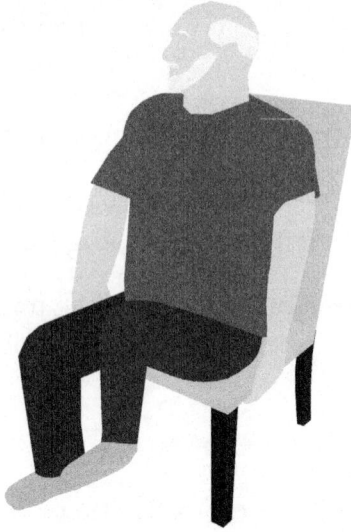

Hip Marching

This exercise targets the hips and thighs and improves flexibility.

1. Maintain an upright seated position without relying on the chair's backrest. Securely hold on to the sides of the chair.

2. Lift your left leg as far as comfortable with your knee bent. In a controlled movement, place your foot down.

3. Repeat with the opposite leg.

4. Do five lifts with each leg.

ANKLE STRETCHES

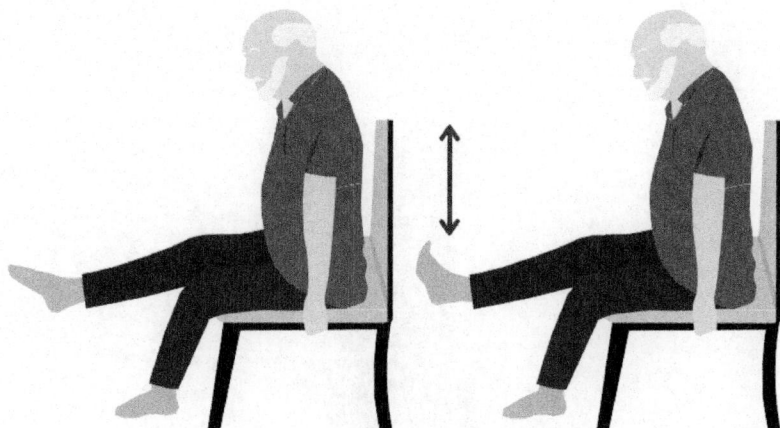

Ankle Stretches

This stretch will improve ankle flexibility.

1. Sitting upright, hold on to the side of the chair. Extend your left leg, lifting your foot off the floor.

2. Keep your leg straight and raised and point your toes away from you.

3. Slowly point your toes back towards you.

4. Try two sets of five stretches with each foot.

ARM RAISES

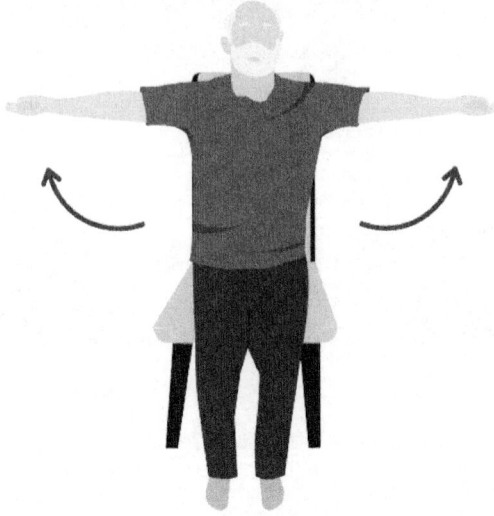

Arm Raises

This exercise helps to build shoulder strength.

1. Sit upright with your arms relaxed by your side.

2. With palms forward, raise both arms out to the side, and up as far as is comfortable.

3. Gently return to the starting position.

4. Keep your shoulders relaxed and arms straight, without bending them at the elbows.

5. Breathe out as you raise your arms and breathe in as you lower them.

6. Repeat five times.

NECK ROTATIONS

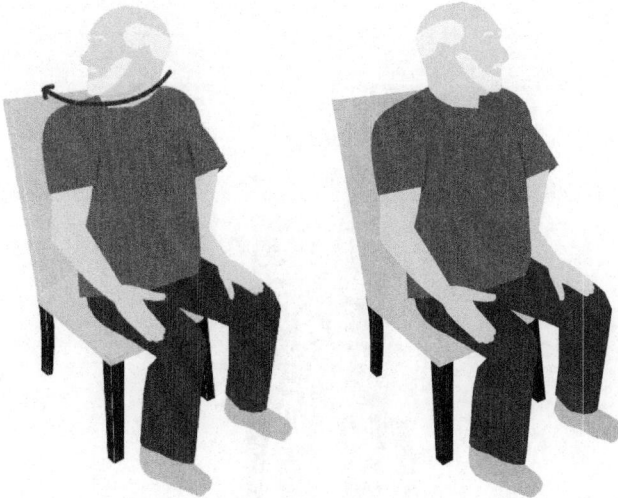

Neck Rotations

This stretch is beneficial for improving neck mobility and flexibility.

1. Sit upright with your shoulders down and relaxed. Look straight ahead.

2. Gently rotate your head towards your left shoulder as far as it feels comfortable. Hold for 5 seconds then return to the starting position.

3. Repeat on the right.

4. Do three rotations on each side.

UPPER BODY TWIST

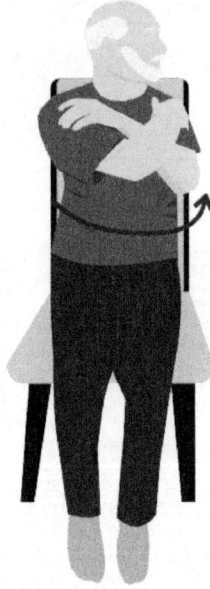

*Upper Body
Twists*

This stretching will improve and maintain flexibility in your upper back.

1. Sit up straight with your feet flat on the floor.

2. Cross your arms and hold onto your shoulders.

3. Without moving your hips or the rest of the lower body, use your upper body to turn to the left as far as is comfortable. Hold for 5 seconds.

4. Repeat on the right side.

5. Do it five times on each side.

CHEST STRETCH

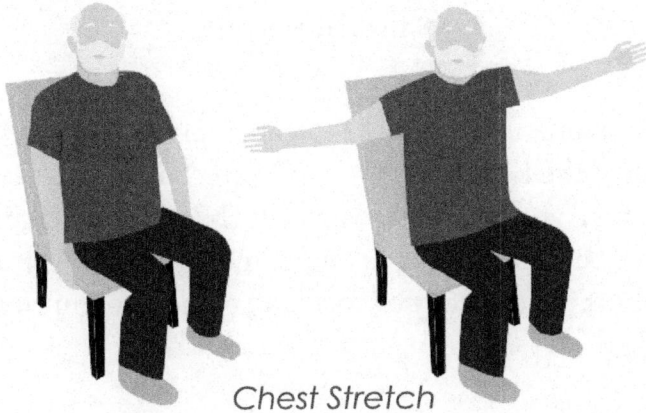

Chest Stretch

This stretch is good for posture and also a good reverse stretch for the upper body stretch.

1. Sit upright without leaning on the back of the chair. Pull your shoulders back and down. Hold on to the chair sides if needed. Straighten your arms out to the side.

2. Gently lift and push your chest forward up until you feel a stretching sensation across your chest.

3. Hold for 5 to 10 seconds and repeat five times.

4. Repeat this routine any time of the day or even before your chair yoga routine to loosen your muscles and get a good stretch to your body.

For breath is life, and if you breathe well you will live long on the earth.

— Sanskrit Proverb

Breath is one more thing you can control, and it will help you control the benefits you reap from chair yoga. The good news is that you're finally ready to begin your chair yoga sequences because you have all the mental and physical tools that support it. Let's start by focusing on how to improve your mobility.

Make a Difference with Your Review

Unlock the Power of Giving

"We can't help everyone, but everyone can help someone"
~ Ronald Reagan

If you are getting value from this book, please allow others access to the information by writing a review. We want to make Ultimate Chair Yoga for Seniors Over 60 accessible to everyone who needs it. Your review could help:

- one more person gain their independence back
- one more person have new meaning in their life
- one more person achieve more flexibility and mobility

Simply scan the QR code or click the link below to leave your review. Thank you!

CHAPTER 6

Stay Mobile With 10-Minute Exercises

We have looked at preparing our space, mind, and body. We have looked at warmups, cooldowns, the mind-body connection, and the dietary changes we should make to support our chair yoga practice. In other words, we have completed all the steps we need for the best possible chair yoga practice. In this chapter, we will look at our first chair yoga sequence, which focuses on improving. About 85% of people over 60 have a normal gait (the manner/the way you walk), while only 18% of people over 85 can say the same (Billot et al., 2020). It is alarming how rapidly our body declines as we age after 60. While there is no way to fully reverse it, practicing chair yoga to improve mobility as early as possible may delay the loss and limits. Let's first understand why mobility changes as we age.

Understanding Mobility

What Is Mobility?

Mobility is about how you move, specifically how well your joints move through their full range of motion (ACE, Megala, 2022). Achieving full joint mobility is vital for sustaining a high quality of life and preserving independence.

Everyday tasks like walking up and down the stairs or bending down to tie your shoelaces are everyday proof of your mobility.

Why Is Mobility so Important, Especially as We Age?

With age, our bodies can start losing mobility, our joints become stiff, and the activities we used to do with ease start becoming more challenging. Gradually, a lack of mobility can lead to decreased independence and increased falls, disease, loss of function, and even death (National Institute on Aging, 2020b). Losing mobility can seriously affect your quality of life.

Losing balance and coordination are also factors that, albeit indirectly, affect mobility. They can cause a serious hindrance in how we move and interact with the world around us, often needing support, essentially losing independence. There are several reasons why you may lose your balance and coordination, including:

- Inner ear problems. When the labyrinth, a part of the inner ear responsible for balance, becomes inflamed, it causes a condition called labyrinthitis. This condition can cause vertigo and imbalance and can be caused by certain ear diseases and infections.

- Alcohol. Inner ear challenges can also come from having alcohol in the blood, causing dizziness and balance problems.

- Other medical conditions. Certain chronic conditions, such as diabetes and heart disease or vision, thyroid, or nerve problems can also cause balance problems.

Since mobility is directly connected to your physical independence and quality of life, it can be incredibly important to maintain it as we age. But given the drastic change in mobility between the ages of 60 and 85, it makes sense to examine what it is that causes us to lose mobility.

Why Do We Lose Mobility With Age?

Age-Related Loss of Mobility

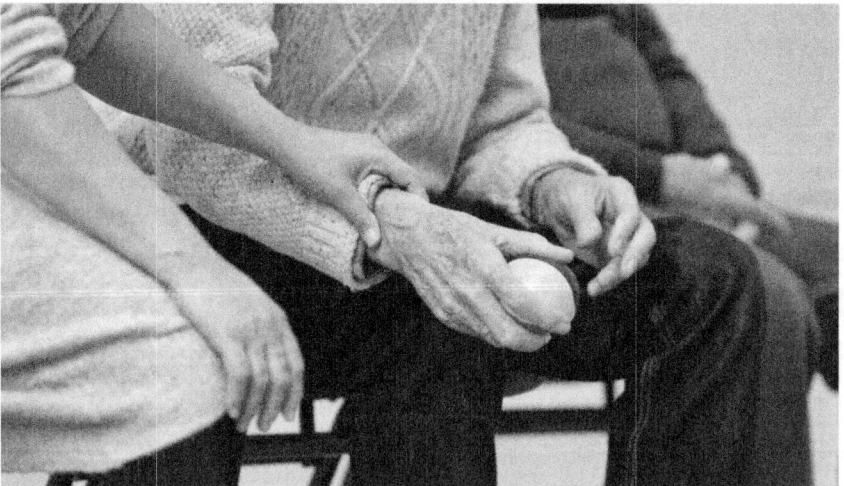

Some decreases in mobility are just a part of getting older. As we lose collagen, a structure that holds water and provides fluid and suppleness to joints, it becomes harder for joints to access their full range of motion.

Also, as we age, certain conditions, such as hypertension, heart disease, diabetes, and arthritis are also associated with mobility loss (Kujala et al., 2019). Sarcopenia, also known as age-related muscle loss, can also contribute to the drop in mobility.

Bone health and density can also affect mobility. With age, we experience a reduction in bone density, which weakens our bones and, in turn, may elevate the risk of fractures. In addition, the cartilage that lines our joints becomes thinner, and the lubricating (synovial) fluid, which protects joints and ensures smooth movement, reduces. This can cause great discomfort. Joints also become stiffer due to more rigid ligaments and tendons and muscle tone and bone strength are reduced. This can significantly affect our body's mobility.

It may seem like balance and coordination loss result from reduced mobility but it is a two-way street. Falls and lack of coordination can happen for various reasons including certain chronic conditions which cause reduced mobility along with an increased uncertainty in movement and a confidence knock. Many active seniors have found increased stability through tai chi, which utilizes slow, deliberate movements that improve range of motion and leg strength. It also increases flexibility and reflexes. When practicing tai chi, you develop the ability on how to shift your body weight in a controlled manner that helps maintain stability, strengthen your muscles, and keep you upright. Some changes at the cellular level in our connective tissue can also cause mobility loss.

We discuss some of these below:

- Changes in how our bodies respond to infection and inflammation are due to changes in hormones, protein development, and growth factors.

- A reduction in the capacity that various cells in our bodies have to grow and divide.

- Slower repair and regeneration of connective tissues.

- As cells age, their function may diminish and become irregular, marked by an increase in pigments and fatty substances within the cell. The accumulation of waste products in tissues, and other associated complications can also occur.

- Altered control of apoptosis (programmed cell death).

Along with a reduction in synovial fluid, joints can also start feeling stiffer and less flexible because ligaments tend to shorten and lose some flexibility.

Whereas the aging in cells and tissues means that cartilage and joints are more susceptible to damage. This process can also lead to an imbalance between catabolic and anabolic activity, caused by the production of inflammatory substances in the cartilage and neighboring joint tissues. This imbalance, along with the joint cell's decreased power of growth and regeneration, causes the secretion of certain chemicals, which cause inflammation.

Synovial fluid contains a large concentration of hyaluronic acid, which gives it the viscosity it needs to act as a sufficient joint lubricant, naturally cushioning joints and surrounding tissues. As you age, the size of the hyaluronic acid molecules in joints diminishes, reducing its effectiveness in performing this vital function.

There are plenty of age-related reasons for mobility loss that cannot be helped and are reasonably out of our control. But there is one significant one we can control and even reverse to an extent. That reason is lack of use.

Repetitive motions that become ingrained in our muscles are another culprit for loss of mobility. One very common example of this is typing on a keyboard. Typing can shorten the muscles in the front chest. If you're also hunched forward—a common posture when sitting at a desk—then you are over-stretching the muscles in your back.

With time, if you continue in this posture, some of your muscles can become chronically shorted while others become chronically elongated. The danger is that this can cause wear and tear on joints that, long-term can lead to chronic pain.

Additionally, sitting at your desk for long periods at a time can reduce your movement. Without regular physical activity, your joints are not conditioned to move through their full range of motions, which is a significant cause of mobility loss in older adults.

So Then How Do We Maintain Mobility As We Grow Older?

We can start by exercising and moving our bodies more to maintain mobility from a younger age. But if you have missed that train, fear not! Everybody starts somewhere, and you can start at whatever health position you are in. With time and consistent efforts, you can still significantly improve your mobility and stability, however old you may be.

Possibly, the best way to achieve this is to avoid a sedentary lifestyle. We don't have to go from the couch straight to a marathon, but based on our physical abilities, the key is to maintain a relatively active life. Some steps we can easily incorporate are:

- **Get regular exercise:** A majority of people know that exercise is associated with a healthier heart and a decreased risk of various diseases, including cancer and diabetes. Regular physical activity also helps maintain your mobility and stay limber. It's one of the most effective ways to enhance your overall well-being during retirement.

- **Eat a balanced diet:** Nutrition also plays a vital role in preserving mobility.

- Eating well can even reduce the impact and the damage to your body caused by falling. Lean protein paired with fruits and vegetables is believed to be the cornerstone of a healthy diet (World Health Organization).

- **Incorporate strength training:** There is mounting evidence that shows strength training improves and maintains core strength. Building muscle mass is another safeguard for staying mobile.

- **See the doctor regularly:** If you don't have one, it's important to find a primary care doctor you feel comfortable with and see them regularly. This proactive approach can help treat small problems as they arise before they become big ones.

While these are some of the more body-focused steps, they can sometimes be daunting, especially when we are just starting out. Staying active does not have to be so complicated, it can be simple things like doing daily chores like cooking, cleaning, or walking the dog. Things you can easily incorporate into your life that naturally involve movement and utilize the different muscles and joints.

Stretching is another way to maintain the lubrication of your joints. Stretching exercises that specifically target the shoulders, spine, hips, and calves can combat chronic stiffness that contributes to mobility loss in older adults. Both dynamic and bend-and-hold types of stretching are great opportunities to move your joints in ways that might not otherwise occur or engage joints that might otherwise be inactive.

Whichever way you bend and stretch, focus on challenging yourself without experiencing pain. Overexerting during stretches can damage your joints and contribute to injury. The objective is to feel a gentle, enjoyable stretch in your muscles. If something doesn't feel good, listen to what your body is saying and reduce the stretch or avoid it altogether.

Cardio exercise helps to create a healthy cardiovascular system, which encourages longevity and mobility. Zumba, kickboxing, and swimming are a few of the ways to help you stay active while having fun at the same time. Senior-focused low-impact cardio exercise sessions can help seniors focus on specific mobility issues.

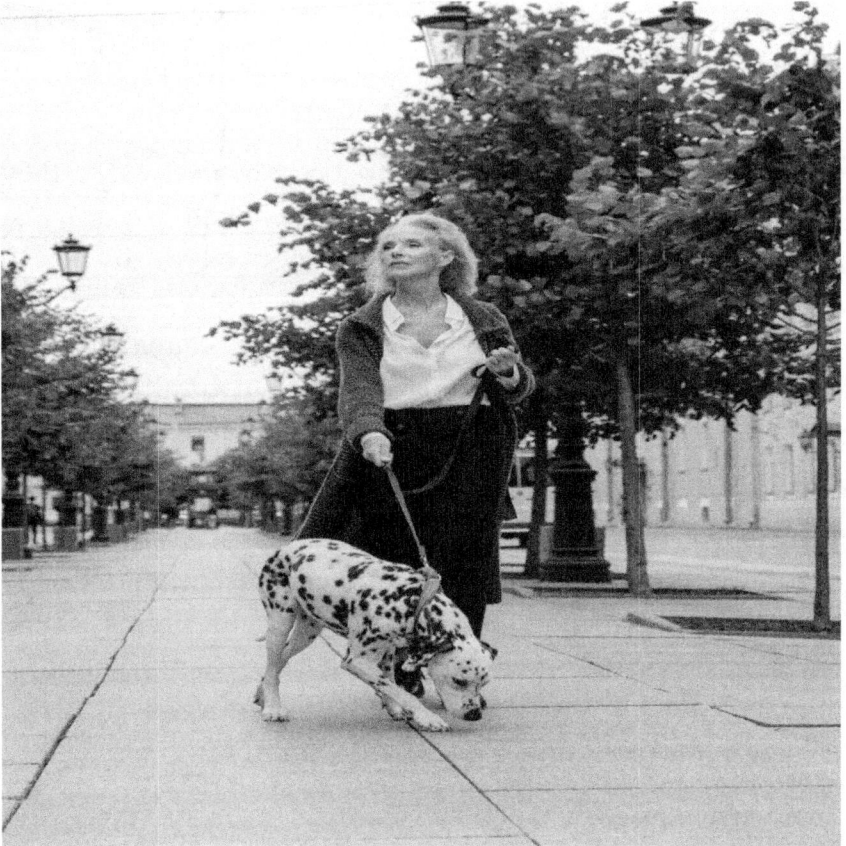

Issues With Balance and Balancing Disorders

If you have a balance disorder, you may experience symptoms such as:

- dizziness or vertigo

- falling or feeling as though you are about to fall

- experiencing dizziness or staggering when walking

- feeling faint

- difficulty focusing or blurred vision

- feeling disoriented or lightheaded

Other symptoms might include nausea and vomiting, diarrhea, changes in heart rate, blood pressure, and feelings of fear, anxiety, or panic. These may all be temporary or recurrent, depending on the person and the symptom. Longer recurring symptoms can lead to fatigue and depression.

There are some specific head and body movement exercises that can help treat some balance disorders. If you struggle with your balance or have a balance disorder, discuss it with your physical therapist or other trained professional, as they will be able to help you with exercises specific to your symptoms and body.

Balance issues can be caused by both high and low blood pressure. In the case of high blood pressure can be managed by reducing salt (sodium) intake, adopting a healthier diet, and exercising to achieve a healthier weight. If low blood pressure is the cause, drink plenty of water and herbal tea. Additionally, it's wise to avoid alcohol, caffeine, and carbonated beverages. Some general ways to address these issues include being cautious with movements, such as avoiding sudden changes in position and working on posture.

It is always advisable to speak with your doctor before making any changes to your diet or activity level, especially in the case of serious balance disorders. Taking specific precautions to prevent falls, such as avoiding walking in the dark, refraining from wearing high heels as they can cause imbalance, and opting for nonskid, rubber-soled, low-heeled shoes instead, can also be beneficial. Finally, avoiding walking on stairs or floors in socks or shoes with smooth soles can help prevent slipping.

In Chapter 1, we explored how chair yoga benefits mobility, flexibility, balance, and coordination. Now, we understand that it also incorporates elements of light cardio, stretching, and strength training. So just follow the sequence for ten minutes daily to access these benefits.

Chair Yoga For Mobility

Our first chair yoga sequence, which focuses on mobility, is a ten-minute sequence with a total of ten steps.

UJJAYI BREATHING

This is a great starting pose.

A. Maintain an upright position at the edge of your seat and place your hands on your waist.

B. Inhale deeply through the nose, allowing your sides and abdomen to expand, and then exhale slowly.

C. Repeat for ten breaths.

Expanding through your waist can sound unusual in the beginning but if you just focus on how your chest and abdomen area is moving during inhalation, you can consciously ensure that your sides and abdomen are expanding.

CHAIR PIGEON

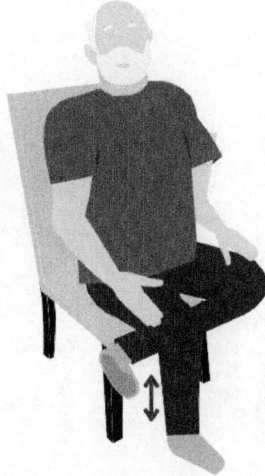

Chair Pigeon

A. Sit upright with your back positioned away from the back of the chair and face forward.

B. Gently lift your left ankle and place it on top of your right knee or thigh. If you have difficulty bringing your ankle to your knee, just use your hand to assist.

C. Inhale deeply, flex your left foot slightly and bend forward upon the exhale.

D. After several deep breaths in the forward position, return to sitting up straight.

E. Gently transition to the other side, so your right ankle rests on your left thigh or knee, and then repeat the preceding steps.

F. Repeat this a few times as your body allows.

EAGLE ARMS

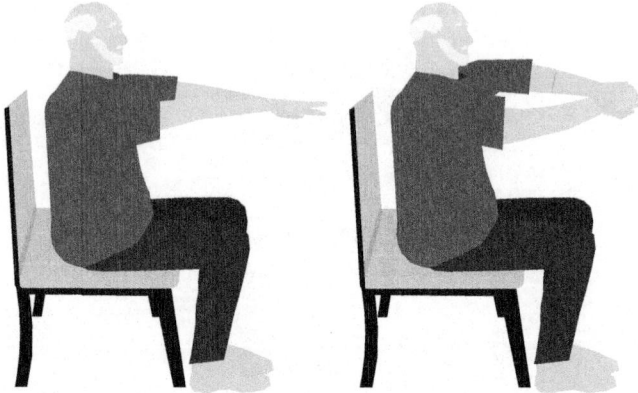

Eagle Arms

A. Maintain an upright seated position and stretch your arms straight out in front of you so that they are in line with your shoulders.

B. Cross your left arm over your right arm so that they cross over at the elbows.

C. Bend your elbows keeping your forearms together.

D. Interlace your fingers and raise your elbows slightly, arching your back a bit. Hold this position for several deep breaths.

E. Upon completion, switch to your right arm over your left arm.

F. Repeat this a few times as your body allows.

SEATED MOUNTAIN POSE

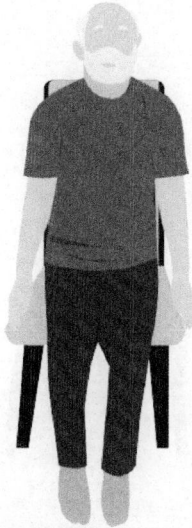

Seated Mountain

A. Begin this pose by sitting on the front edge of your chair with a straight back and an engaged core.

B. Bend your knees at 90-degree angles, ensuring they are positioned above your ankles, with a slight gap between your knees.

C. Inhale slowly and roll your shoulders downward upon exhaling. Focus on lengthening your spine and extending your feet into the floor like the roots of a tree.

D. Activate your abdominal muscles and hold your arms down at your sides with some tension.

E. Hold the pose for several deep breaths.

CHAIR SPINAL TWIST

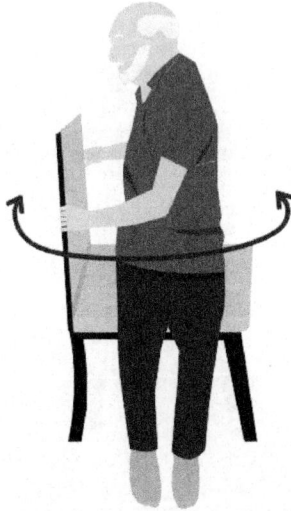

Chair Spinal twists

A. Sit sideways in your chair with your knees aligned over the right side of the chair and the back of the chair next to your right arm.

B. Make sure your back is straight, and your body is apart from the back of the chair.

C. Grasp the back of the chair with both hands, breathe in, then slowly turn your body toward the back of the chair while exhaling.

D. Hold this position for several breaths before returning to the original position.

E. After completing this pose, switch to the opposite side of the chair so your knees are positioned over the left side of the chair, and the chair's back is next to your left arm.

WARRIOR I POSE

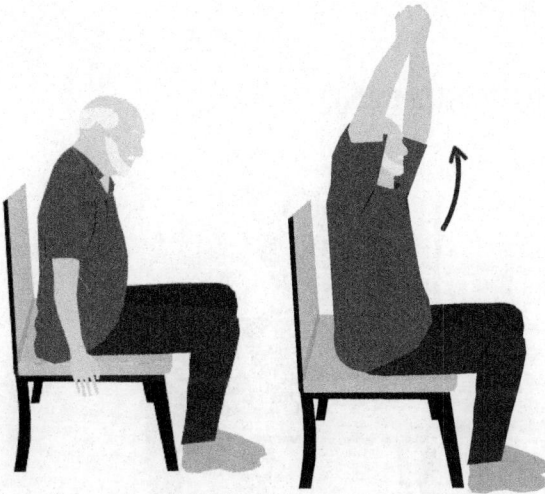

Warrior I Pose

This pose takes a Seated Mountain pose and adds in arm movement to get the blood flowing.

A. As you inhale, bring your arms out to the sides and straighten them up over your head.

B. Hold them here for five deep breaths. You can interlock your fingers for added support.

C. Make sure to keep your head level with the ground and your eyes gazing forward, not up, your back is straight.

D. Bring your arms back down to your sides as you exhale.

E. As you get more comfortable you can straddle the chair and move into a standing pose. You'll still have most of your body weight on the chair so you can worry less about balance.

SEATED FORWARD BEND

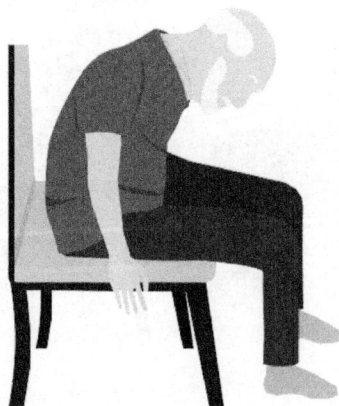

Seated
Forward Bend

A. Start in the Seated Mountain pose.

B. Inhale and sit up tall, then exhale and slowly bend forward over your thighs.

C. Keep your arms at your sides to engage your core muscles for added difficulty or place your hands on your thighs and then shin bones as you bend forward. This will help make the movement easier and offer you greater control in case you need to take a break or back out of the pose.

D. Stay in the forward bend position for three to five breaths and then slowly return to the Seated Mountain pose.

SEATED SIDE ANGLE POSE

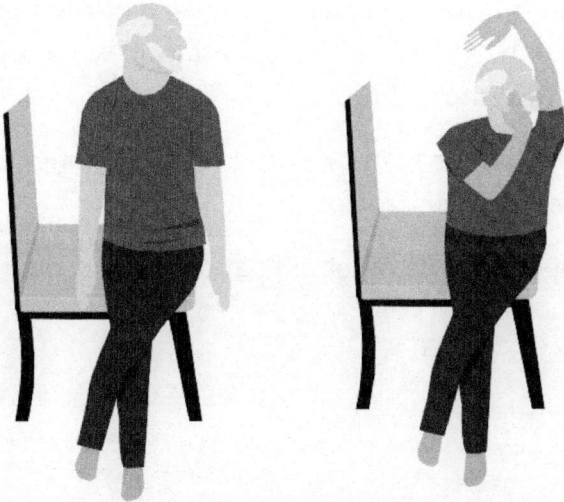

Seated Side Angle Pose

This is a more advanced chair yoga pose and should only be completed if you are able to support half of your body weight off the chair.

A. Start with your right thigh and buttocks on the chair. Maintain a sideways orientation.

121

B. Your left leg should be at a 90-degree angle, not on the chair. Keep your right foot directly beneath your right knee. Your left knee can be over your right foot for the easiest way of doing this pose. For added difficulty, you can move your left leg straight out or even slightly behind you.

C. While your right leg is facing sideways, turn your hips so that they face the front of the chair.

D. Bring your arms straight out to your sides and slowly lengthen directly over your right leg. Place your right elbow on your right thigh.

E. Gently raise your left arm over your left ear pointing your left hand in the direction of your right leg but toward the ceiling.

F. Look under your arm toward the ceiling and hold for a few breaths.

G. Repeat on the other side and do the sequence three to four times.

SUN SALUTATION ARMS POSE

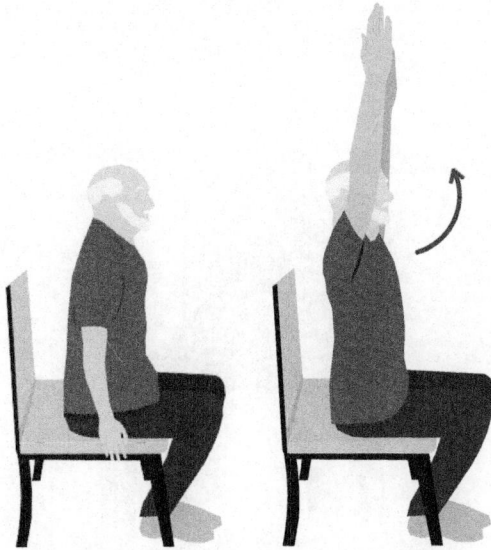

Sun Salutation Arms Pose

This helps lengthen the spine and reduce tension in the shoulders and neck.

A. Sit tall, breathe in, and lift your arms up, pressing your palms overhead.

B. On an exhale, float the arms back down to your sides.

C. Repeat five times.

GODDESS WITH A TWIST

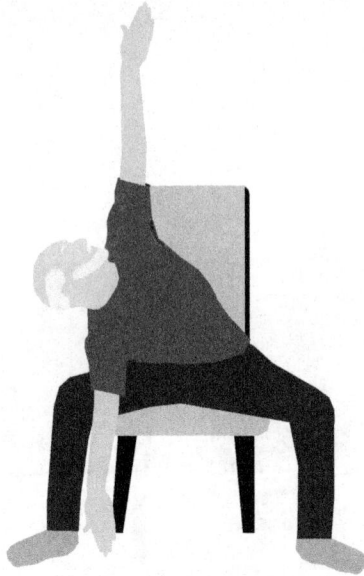

*Coddess With
A Twist*

A. Place your legs wide apart and point your toes out.

B. Place your right arm inside your right leg, reaching toward the floor.

C. Elevate your left arm up to the ceiling and look towards your left palm.

D. Hold for five breaths, then repeat on the opposite side.

This makes up your first chair yoga sequence. It focuses on moving otherwise unused muscles and joints of the body as well as stretching your body.

Mobility is one of the foundations of our prosperity.

— Franz Müntefering

Increasing your mobility and range of motion is the first step toward physical independence. You enjoy life more when you can move around without worrying about stumbles or falls. Your balance also matters, and it's connected to your mobility. Practice your 10-minute mobility sequence while alternating the sequences with the next two for strength and pain management. Doing one sequence a day will help you exercise each major point once in three days. Next, let's uncover the chair yoga workouts designed to build muscle strength and minimize the risk of falling further.

CHAPTER 7

Build Muscles and Strength to Prevent Falls

In this section, we will be looking at the next chair yoga sequence which focuses on building strength in your muscles to protect you from injuries and falls. It will also strengthen the thinner fibers in your body which might get ignored otherwise during normal activity.

The decline of muscle mass typically begins in your 30s and 40s but speeds up after 65, and you could lose up to 8% of your muscle mass every decade in your senior years (Cleveland Clinic, 2022). While mobility is extremely important as we age, so is muscle strength. And it's time to focus on your muscles to help your aging journey. Before we dive into the exercises to increase our muscle strength, let's first find out more about why this muscle loss happens and what we can do to avoid this loss apart from exercising.

Why Do We Lose Muscles With Age?

Our muscles start feeling weaker with age, reducing both our strength and energy. This muscle loss is called sarcopenia and after 30, it can result in a loss of 3% to 5% of muscle mass per decade. Most men can lose as much as 30% of their muscle mass over their lifetime (Harvard Health Publishing, 2016).

The increased loss of mobility and muscle strength may increase your risk of falls and fractures. Those diagnosed with sarcopenia are 2.3 times more likely to suffer a low-trauma fracture, such as a broken hip or wrist from a fall (American Society for Mineral Research, 2015). Even though muscle loss occurs, it is still possible for both men and women to increase muscle mass as they age (Harvard Health Publishing, 2016).

Reduced Muscle Size and Strength

In addition to weakened strength and muscle fibers, muscle loss also reduces our exercise tolerance. This is caused by several factors working together, including:

- Muscle fibers reduce in quantity and undergo shrinkage.

- Muscle tissue undergoes replacement at a slower pace, and lost muscle tissue is substituted with tough, fibrous tissue.

- Alterations in the nervous system cause muscles to have reduced tone and the ability to contract.

Hormonal Changes

Hormonal changes also affect the muscle composition in the body, with age, the following changes in endocrine function result in sarcopenia:

- increased insulin resistance

- decreased growth hormone

- vitamin D deficiency

- increased parathyroid hormone

These changes can affect both men and women; however, different hormones cause different changes, so we will discuss them separately.

Hormonal Changes in Men

For men, the natural decline in testosterone, the hormone essential for stimulating protein synthesis and muscle growth, can be a contributing factor to sarcopenia.

No matter our age, the best way to build muscle mass, is through progressive resistance training (PRT). This form of training involves gradually increasing your workout volume either by increasing weight, reps, or sets as your strength and endurance improve. By constantly challenging yourself, you not only build muscle mass and strength, you also strengthen your mental capacity and endurance.

A recent study examining 49 research studies of men aged 50 to 83 participating in Progressive Resistance Training (PRT) found that, on average, subjects achieved a 2.4-pound increase in lean body mass (Harvard Health Publishing, 2016).

You may be curious about supplements. Some studies have shown that supplemental testosterone can add lean body mass or muscle in older men, but there can also be adverse effects (Harvard Health Publishing, 2016). It's worth noting that the FDA has yet to approve these supplements specifically for increasing muscle mass in men. Any supplemental hormone ingestion can carry some risk and should not be done without a consultation with your healthcare provider.

Hormonal Changes in Women

Menopause is one of the most significant changes that women go through as they age. During this natural aging process, women experience hormonal changes in particular, a decline in estrogen levels. Estradiol, the most potent estrogen hormone, plays a vital role in regulating the menstrual cycle and is responsible for the development and upkeep of the reproductive system. Interestingly, the skeletal muscle possesses specific estradiol receptors at the fiber levels, which means that estradiol can promote muscle regeneration and contribute to muscle health.

The menopausal transition is not only associated with a decline in estradiol levels, but also with an increased tendency for fat deposition and decreased bone density, muscle mass, and muscle strength.

Changes in Muscle Fiber

From 25 onward, the total number of muscle fibers starts reducing significantly, which is most likely due to decreases in total fiber numbers.

With age, muscle fibers decrease in area, and fiber number. Studies suggest a connection between both the decline in muscle quality and balance coordination among older adults, and a decrease in muscle fiber size and number (Physiopedia, 2019b).

This muscle fiber loss is due to a loss of motor neurons. As we age, muscle fiber regeneration slows down, therefore reducing the number of muscle fibers. Data indicates that a 60-year-old has approximately 25-50% fewer motor neurons than a 20-year-old (Bunn JA, 2012).

Effects of Muscle Loss

It is natural to think that loss of strength or increase in frailty, is a direct consequence of muscle loss. This is absolutely true, but there are other effects of this muscle loss as well.

- The decline in testosterone levels in men and estrogen levels in women is associated not only with loss in muscle mass but also an increase in visceral fat. Visceral fat is located around the abdomen region, which is seen as the most dangerous type of fat (Paul Frysh, 2021). An excess of visceral fat can affect all the vital organs, as most of them reside in the abdominal region.

- The decrease of lean body mass reduces function, and the loss of approximately 40% of lean body mass is fatal (R Roubenoff, 2001).

- This has been attributed to a reduction of muscle size as well as a reduction in satellite cells — a stem cell that lies adjacent to skeletal muscle fiber and plays a vital role in muscle growth, regeneration, and repair — mitochondrial numbers and elasticity.

- Sarcopenia has a major effect on function in all activities of daily living, contributing to reduced gait speed, falls, and fractures. The combination of osteoporosis and sarcopenia results in the frailty that frequently occurs among seniors.

How Can We Prevent Muscle Loss?

Loss of muscle strength can be detrimental to your independence, mobility, energy levels, and even confidence. While you may not be able to completely reverse all the muscle mass that has been lost, you can definitely gain back enough of it to make your life easier and more comfortable. The question is, how do we do that? Let's explore.

Diet

What you eat can significantly influence how much muscle mass, strength, and endurance you sustain in your senior years. Proper nutrition is essential in building muscle mass. The saying "abs are made in the kitchen" is true. And while we don't need to go to the extent of trying to get 6-pack abs, the fundamental concept of monitoring your diet for muscle gain still applies. One food group that is essential for building muscle strength is proteins. Protein is broken down into amino acids by our bodies, which are then utilized in muscle construction.

However, aging men and women commonly face a decrease in their bodies' capability to break down and synthesize protein. Therefore, like PRT, older individuals should aim for higher protein intake in their diet. A recent study proposes a daily ingestion of 1 to 1.3 grams (g) of protein per kilogram of body weight for older adults (Harvard Health Publishing, 2016). For instance, a 175-pound man would need about 79 g to 103 g a day. Ideally, you should divide your protein intake equally over your daily meals to maximize muscle protein synthesis. A high-protein diet along with exercise is key to gaining the muscle mass we have lost over the years.

There are many ways to cover the required protein goals in a high-protein diet. The best protein sources are animal products, as they offer the proper ratios of all the essential amino acids. However, try to avoid red and processed meat, which have high levels of saturated fat and additives. You can instead opt for healthier choices, such as lean chicken or salmon, plain Greek yogurt, skim milk, and cooked beans.

Natural foods are the best sources of proteins but if you are struggling to reach the required amount of protein necessary for your body, you can incorporate supplements like protein powders. Protein powders typically offer around 30 g of protein per scoop and can be easily added into meals like oatmeal, shakes, and yogurt.

To maximize muscle growth and improve recovery, one recommendation is to have a meal or drink with a carbohydrate-to-protein ratio of about three-to-one or four-to-one within 30 minutes following your workout (Harvard Health Publishing, 2016). For example, a good choice is chocolate milk, 8 ounces of which has about 22 g of carbs and 8 g of protein.

Building muscle isn't solely about strength, you also need power. Muscle power, which reflects how quickly and efficiently you move, is more connected to your daily activities and physical function than just muscular strength. Your legs and lower body are more responsible for mobility so it is a good idea to increase muscle strength in this area. Common ways to test and improve muscle power for your lower body could be trying to rise quickly from a seated position or pushing off each step of the stairs as quickly as possible. It does not have to be in every activity, but you should start trying little by little and be more aware of such movements.

Physical Activity

One of the most effective methods for preserving muscle mass is regular physical activity. Engaging in exercise can reduce the effects of sarcopenia, potentially even reversing some of its symptoms. For older adults, preserving muscle mass and function is crucial for maintaining independence and enjoying later life.

Low-impact activities like walking, resistance training, gentle aerobics, yoga, and tai chi offer many benefits to the body.

Ideally, our exercise routines should cover the "fabs" acronym, focusing on flexibility, aerobic fitness, balance, and strength to maintain optimal health.

Low-impact joint-releasing exercises, which gently flex and tone the muscles, as well as work the ligaments and tendons, can also be very helpful. These exercises are beneficial for enhancing flexibility and mobility throughout the body, particularly in areas like the shoulders, wrists, hands, foot flexors, and ankles. The idea behind such physical activity is to cause micro-tears in the muscle, which, when repaired and regenerated, increase the muscle composition and overall bodily strength to endure physical strain.

Yoga is normally safe for people with muscular dystrophy, progressive weakness, and a loss of muscle mass. However, it's important to consult with a doctor beforehand and take any necessary precautions. With over 30 different types of muscular dystrophy, varying in severity, progression, and affected muscles, individualized treatment plans are critical for safety and effectiveness. Chair yoga can be especially beneficial as it minimizes the risk while providing a lot of the same benefits that regular yoga can give you.

Chair Yoga for Strength

It is finally time to look at the ten-minute chair yoga for strength, which includes ten different asanas (poses) that you can do on the chair.

MOUNTAIN POSE WITH CAT-COW

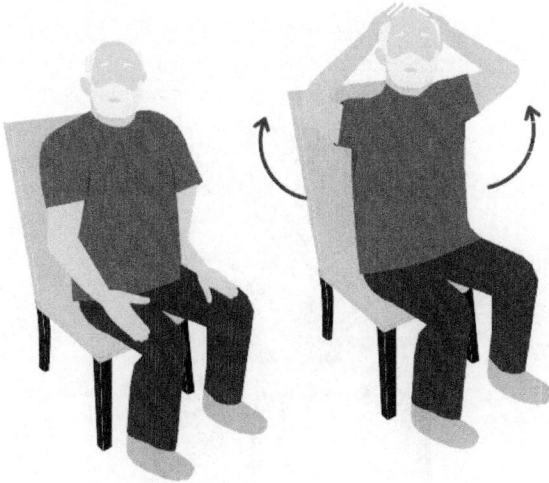

Mountain Pose with Cat-Cow

The goal of Mountain Pose is a strong, upright posture. For this, follow the steps:

A. Sit toward the front of your chair.

B. Set your feet and knees hip-width apart, and place your hands on your thighs or allow them to fall down by your sides.

C. Reach the crown of your head toward the ceiling to lengthen your spine.

D. Allow your shoulders to relax away from your ears.

E. Look forward, keeping your chin parallel to the floor and some space at the back of your neck.

BHARADVAJA'S TWIST

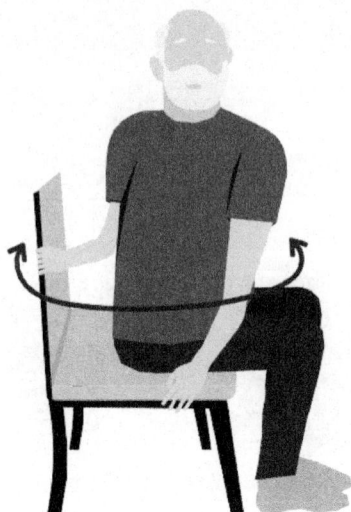

Bharadvaja's Twist

A. Begin in Mountain Pose, sitting toward the front edge of your seat.

B. Inhale and lengthen your spine.

C. On an exhalation, twist to the right, keeping your hip points facing forward and turning from your waist and shoulders.

D. Bring your left hand to the outside of your right thigh for gentle leverage, and reach your right arm back and hold the back of the chair for stability.

E. Breathe in this pose, gently deepening your twist if that feels comfortable for you on each exhalation.

F. When you are ready, release your hands and unwind to return to Mountain Pose.

G. Repeat on the opposite side.

COW FACE POSE

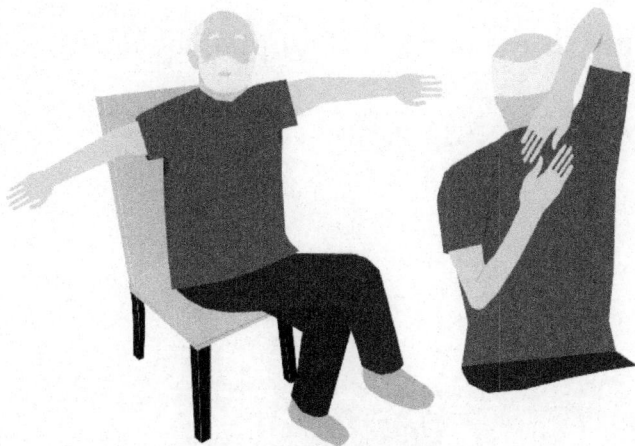

Cow Face Pose

A. From Mountain Pose, bring your feet and legs together.

B. Lift your right leg and cross it over your left thigh.

C. Stretch your arms out to the sides parallel to the floor.

D. Reach up with your left hand and bring your bicep in line with your ear, then bend your elbow and reach your hand toward the back of your neck.

E. Rotate your right arm internally so that your palm faces behind you.

F. Bend your right elbow and bring the back of your hand toward your spine.

G. Reach down with your left hand and up with your right, inching your hands along your spine toward one another. Your fingers may meet, but it's fine if they don't.

H. Unwind and repeat on the opposite side.

EXTENDED TRIANGLE POSE

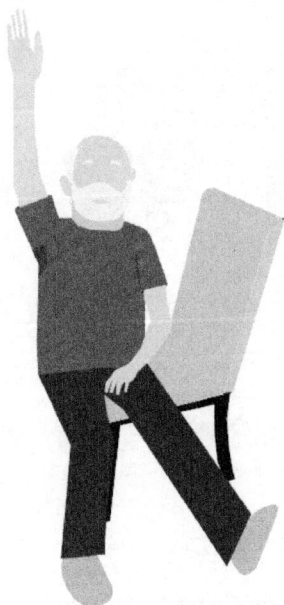

Extended Triangle Pose

A. From Mountain Pose shift to the left side of your chair so that your left buttock is on the very edge of your seat.

B. Plant your feet on the floor with your knees aligned over your ankles.

C. Open your left leg out to the side so that your legs are perpendicular to each other. Straighten your left leg.

D. Inhale, lengthening your spine as you raise your arms and extend them out to the sides parallel to the floor.

E. On an exhale, lean to the left, and bring your left hand to your left leg.

F. Extend your right arm straight up with your palm forward.

G. In this position, you may choose to look forward or turn your head to look up at your right hand. When you are ready, lift your torso back to seated and bring your left leg to meet your right.

H. Shift to the right side of your seat and repeat the pose on the opposite side.

SEATED OVERHEAD STRETCH

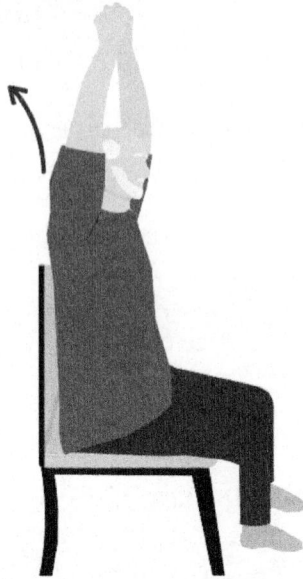

Seated Overhead Stretch

A. Sit tall in a chair with your feet flat on the floor.

B. Reach your arms overhead, interlacing your fingers.

C. Carefully pull your arms back until you feel a stretch in your shoulders and sides.

D. Hold for 5–10 breaths before returning to the starting position.

FIREFLY POSE

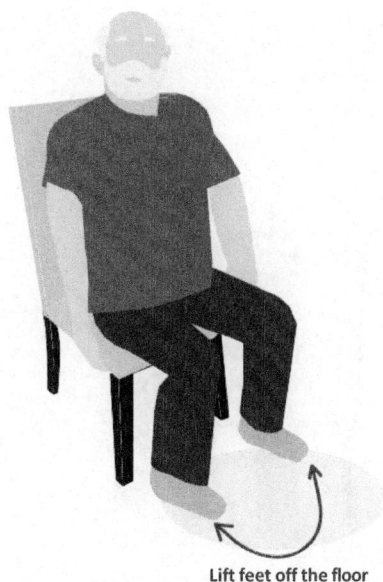

Lift feet off the floor

Firefly Pose

A. From Mountain Pose, open your knees out wide toward the corners of the seat of your chair.

B. Bring your hands to rest on the front edge of the seat.

C. Lengthen your spine, engage your abs, and press your hands strongly into the chair seat, as if you were going to lift your body off the chair in Firefly.

D. Engage your quads to straighten both legs and lift your feet off the floor.

E. Hold for 5-10 breaths before returning to the starting position.

REVERSE WARRIOR POSE

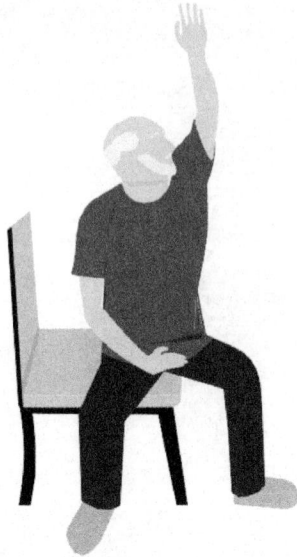

Reverse Warrior Pose

A. From Mountain Pose, shift to the right side of your chair so that your right buttock is off the edge of your seat.

B. Open your left knee out to the side so that your thigh is fully supported by the seat of the chair.

C. Your left foot and knee point left, and your knee is aligned over your ankle.

D. Extend your right leg straight to the right, pressing the outer edge of your foot down and lifting the arch to engage that leg.

E. Inhale, lengthening your spine as you raise your arms and extend them out to the sides parallel to the floor.

F. On an exhale, curve to the right as you reach your left hand toward the ceiling and bring your right hand to your left leg.

G. Look at your left hand in Reverse Warrior.

H. When you are ready, lift your torso back upright. Bend your legs together in the Mountain Pose.

I. Move to the left side of your chair and repeat the pose on the opposite side.

PUPPY POSE

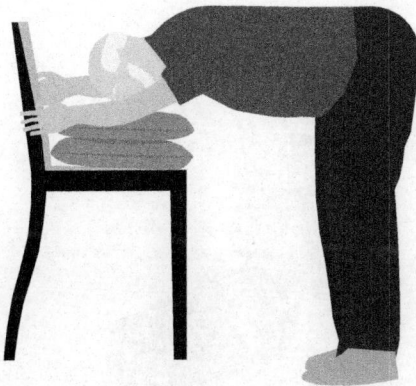

Puppy Pose

A. Stand facing a chair that is set two to three feet in front of you.

B. On an exhale, hinge at your hips and fold forward until your forehead meets the seat of the chair. (You can stack folded blankets or pillows on the chair to raise the height of the seat to meet your head.)

C. Extend your arms forward and rest them on the seat of the chair.

D. For a stronger shoulder opener, arch slightly to place your hands on the back of the chair and press your chest toward the floor to mimic the action of an Extended Puppy Pose.

E. When you are ready, release your hands and press back up to stand.

SEATED WARRIOR II POSE

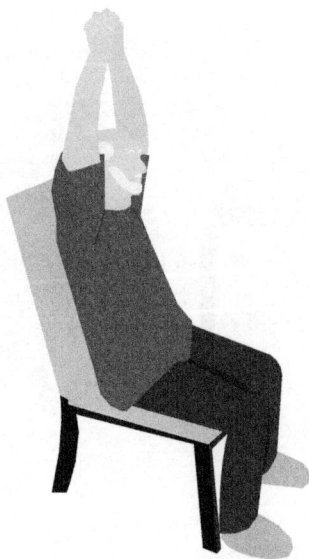

Seated Warrior II Pose

A. Sit tall in a chair with your feet flat on the floor.

B. Stretch your arms out to the sides at shoulder height.

C. Slowly raise your arms overhead and clasp your hands together.

D. Hold for 5-10 breaths before repeating on the other side.

HALF MOON POSE

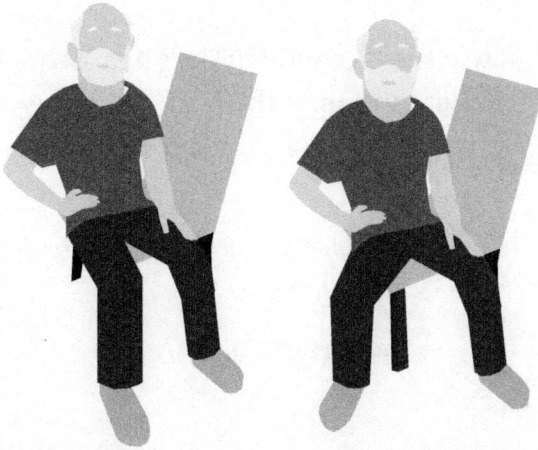

Half Moon Pose

A. From the Extended Triangle, bring your right hand to your hip and turn your head to look at the seat of the chair.

B. Supported by your hand on the chair, move your weight into your left leg and lift your right leg.

C. If you can, bring your thigh parallel to the floor.

D. Turn your chest and hips out to face the right side of the room as if you were trying to stack both hips and shoulders perpendicular to the floor.

E. Make sure your right knee and toes are also facing right.

F. Keep your right hand on your hip or reach your top hand to the ceiling and turn to look up in Half Moon Pose.

G. Switch the chair to the other side and repeat the pose on the opposite side.

This completes the second chair yoga sequence. It is slightly more challenging than the first one, so use whatever modifications are necessary for your physical level.

Aging is not 'lost youth,' but a new stage of opportunity and strength.

— Betty Friedan

Don't allow weaker muscles or less mass to risk your opportunity to enjoy the golden years. Improving your muscle strength during this time can open your world to opportunities that are much more than expected. It also reduces your risk of falling. Add your 10-minute sequence to your alternate days to see the benefits of strengthening your muscles with chair yoga. Then, you need the final sequence focusing on chronic pain management and joint health.

CHAPTER 8

Manage Pain and Stiffness to Enjoy Life

C hronic pain, stiff joints, and arthritis are common issues in the senior years. We can't stop them from deteriorating, whether with a chronic condition or an old injury. Between 25-85% of seniors suffer from chronic pain (Abdulla et. al. 2013). Pain is not just part of aging, it contributes to functional degeneration, increases the risk of falls and mood disorders, and can cause an increased dependence on institutional care. No one wants to live their life relying on pain medication. But is there a way to manage pain so that it doesn't become a hindrance to our lives? Yes, there is! But first, let's take a look at why joint pain and stiffness are so common among seniors.

Why Do We Suffer from Joint Pain?

The first step in understanding why it happens is to clarify what exactly classifies as joint pain. Joint pain and discomfort can usually be experienced in the places we use most, like hands, feet, hips, knees, or spine. People can either experience constant pain, or it can come and go. It can also manifest in different ways, from stiff, achy, or sore joints to burning, throbbing, or "grating" sensations. Movement and activity also play a role, since joints can often feel stiffer in the morning but loosen up and feel better with the motions of the day. However, too much activity could also make the pain worse. In severe cases, joint pain may change how the joint functions, limiting a person's ability to do basic tasks and having an adverse effect on their quality of life. Treatment should address not just pain but also the impacted activities and functions.

Joint pain tends to affect those who:

- have had previous injuries to a joint.
- repeatedly use and/or overuse a muscle.
- have arthritis or other chronic medical conditions.
- suffer from depression, anxiety, and/or stress.
- are overweight.
- suffer from poor health.
- are middle-aged to older adults.

There are a number of different reasons why joint pain is an issue among the senior population. It can be compounded as many seniors also have previous injuries, chronic medical conditions, and other determining factors that can worsen joint pain. Many of these are because of age-related degeneration but there are other reasons as well. Let's take a closer look at some of them.

Changes to Bone Structure

Our bones are living tissue. As we age, our bone structure changes, resulting in the loss of bone tissue. With a lower bone mass and weaker bones, there is a greater risk that our bones will fracture from a sudden bump or fall.

The reasons why our bones become less dense as we age include:

- An inactive lifestyle can cause bone wastage.

- Hormonal changes. For women, menopause initiates a decrease in bone tissue minerals. In men, diminishing testosterone levels contribute to the eventual onset of osteoporosis.

- As we age, bones gradually lose calcium and other essential minerals.

Changes in the Joints

The bones at our joints do not directly contact each other since they are cushioned by cartilage that lines the joints, synovial membranes surrounding the joint, and lubricating synovial fluid inside the joints. As we discussed earlier, joint movement becomes stiffer and less flexible with age because of a reduction in the synovial fluid, thinner cartilage, and shorter ligaments.

A lack of exercise causes many of these age-related joint changes. By moving and keeping your joints active, you help to keep the fluid moving and keep your joints in good condition. Inactivity is what causes the cartilage to shrink and stiffen, reducing joint mobility.

Health Issues Can Cause Joint Pains

Sometimes overlooked, certain illnesses and chronic health conditions can also cause or increase joint pain in seniors.

Some common conditions that specifically affect joints are:

- Osteoarthritis, a common form of arthritis, happens gradually over time as the protective cartilage between the bones deteriorates. This degeneration leads to painful and stiff joints. Typically, osteoarthritis begins in middle age and progresses slowly.

- Rheumatoid arthritis. It's a chronic condition that causes swelling and pain in the joints. The joints often become deformed—usually occurring in the fingers and wrists.

- Gout. A painful condition where uric acid crystals form in the body and collect in the joint, causing severe pain and swelling. This usually occurs in the big toe. This happens when the kidneys are unable to effectively filter uric acid from the blood.

- Bursitis. Inflammation is caused by overuse of the joints and muscles. It is typically found in joints such as the hip, knee, elbow, or shoulder.

- Tendinitis, marked by inflammation of the tendons, normally affects the elbow, shoulder, or heel, typically resulting from overuse.

- Viral infections, rash, fever, or flu may make joint movement painful.

- Injuries, such as broken bones or sprains.

Osteoarthritis Vs. Rheumatoid Arthritis

Both Osteoarthritis (OA) and Rheumatoid Arthritis (RA) are possibly the most common reasons for joint pain. So, let's examine them further to understand why this is.

RA is an autoimmune disease that develops when your immune system doesn't work how it should. A healthy immune system will attack any bacteria and viruses you are exposed to but with RA, your immune system sees your joints as enemies and launches an attack on them. The symptoms of RA are similar to those of an injury or infectious disease, including tender, warm, swollen, and stiff joints combined with fever, fatigue, and loss of appetite.

On the other hand, OA, which isn't an autoimmune disease, impacts almost 27 million Americans (Michele Jordan, 2021). It develops due to general wear and tear and a breakdown of the cartilage (spongy tissue) between your joints. This causes the bones on either side of the cartilage to change and ache. The cartilage, which provides cushioning between the bone ends within your joints, deteriorates until bone begins to rub against bone. That can be painful!

RA usually attacks the small joints in your hands and feet. one of the things that really sets it apart from OA is that it can cause morning stiffness that may last for some time.

Other RA signs and symptoms may include:

- fatigue

- a fever

- low appetite

- lumps, called rheumatoid nodules that grow under your skin

OA is more likely to affect the joints you use more, like hands, or the ones that support weight like knees. With OA, your main issues are:

- stiffness and pain

- swollen joints

- noises (cracking, grinding) when you move the joint

- joints not working the way they should

Other Chronic Diseases Which May Cause Joint Pain

- **Chronic fatigue syndrome:** (CFS) is a persistent condition that can develop after a viral illness. However, sometimes it can develop on its own, without any obvious trigger. Joint pain is a common symptom of CFS.

- **Lupus:** Also known as systemic lupus erythematosus, Lupus is a chronic autoimmune condition that impacts multiple bodily systems including the joints, skin, kidneys, and brain. It leads to inflammation and tissue damage, particularly in the joints, causing pain. While there is no cure for lupus, treatment is available to help manage symptoms, prevent exacerbations, and protect against organ damage.

- **Psoriatic arthritis (PsA):** This affects about 20% of individuals with psoriasis, resulting in painful inflammation and stiffness in the joints. Treatment strategies for PsA include medication, physical therapy, or exercise, aimed at easing symptoms and halting further joint damage.

Learning all this it is very clear that joint pain shouldn't be taken lightly. While chair yoga can help you manage it, it is very important that you consult a doctor before you start any exercises or new routines to ensure it is safe for your current condition.

Can Joint Pain Be Managed at Home?

Yes. There are a few different ways to manage joint pain on your own, here are some of them.

Supplements

Supplements are often useful in the management of joint pain. Often, we miss out on certain micronutrients in our diet which could be important for our joint health. Adding supplements to your diet can help fill these nutrient deficiencies.

Fish Oil

Foods rich in omega-3 fatty acids, such as salmon, tuna, fish oils, and nuts, support the production of anti-inflammatory chemicals in the body, potentially reducing stiffness and pain. You can also obtain them through supplements.

Glucosamine

These natural substances found in healthy cartilage can protect cartilage and may help stop inflammation. Glucosamine supplements can be created in a lab or made from the cartilage of animals like cows, pigs, or shellfish.

Viscosupplementation

This treatment involves a doctor injecting hyaluronic acid—a naturally occurring substance in joint fluid—into your joint, typically the knee. This fluid lubricates bones, enabling them to move smoothly together. This is an injectable supplement as compared to the other oral ones.

Platelet-Rich Plasma

Doctors can now use your own blood platelets in strong doses to inject back into your joint. These platelets harbor hundreds of proteins known as growth factors, which can help accelerate the healing response in your body. However, there isn't enough evidence yet to determine its effectiveness.

Lifestyle Changes

Certain lifestyle changes can also be supportive in managing pain.

Weight Loss

If you carry some excess weight, it puts extra pressure on your joints, especially knee joints. A study suggests each pound of weight you lose, there is a corresponding reduction in the load on your knee joint by 4 lbs (1.81 kg) (Messier et al., 2005). This means that excess weight can also cause extra wear and tear in your joints and increase the likelihood of joint pain and osteoarthritis.

Sleep

Lack of quality sleep can intensify joint pain, foster feelings of depression, and heighten the likelihood of arthritis-induced disability. It robs your body of necessary rest and restoration time which ensures that all your body parts work well.

Prioritizing sleep starts with good sleep hygiene. This means having a consistent sleep schedule, waking up at relatively the same time each day, and turning off electrical devices — cell phones, laptops, TVs — at least an hour before you go to bed. Incorporating relaxing practices like taking a warm bath, sipping a cup of tea, or meditating can also help improve your sleep.

Quit Smoking

If smoking is part of your daily routine, it would be a good time to reconsider this habit. Smoking causes **a lot** of damage. In addition to having the potential to harm every organ in your body, it can also damage your joints. If you smoke, you're at a higher risk of getting RA and have more severe joint damage if you do. Studies suggest smoking makes the pain from OA worse and can reduce the effectiveness of pain medication in providing relief (Jordan, 2021).

Other Ways to Manage Pain

Topical Treatments

An age-old yet effective treatment involves using ointments or gels that can be rubbed into the skin over the affected area to alleviate pain. These remedies are available over the counter or may be prescribed by a doctor.

Another topical treatment centers on hot and cold therapy. Using an ice pack or heating pad on the affected area for short periods or soaking in a warm bathtub can provide relief.

Low-Impact Cardio

As you know, exercise can help you regain strength and function. Walking, swimming, or other low-impact aerobic exercise is best. If you are used to strenuous workouts or sports activities you may want to scale it back or begin a low-impact workout routine to protect your joints. Gentle stretching exercises will also help. As always, check with your doctor before beginning or continuing any exercise program.

Along with all of these different ways to manage pain, there is one more crucial thing that could make the difference between functioning and non-functioning joints. And that is, moving your joints. If you have joint pain and avoid exercise because you're worried about exacerbating the pain or getting injured, you may be making the problem worse. Exercise is essential for improving joint function and reducing pain. According to the CDC (n.d.), the best results are achieved with 30 minutes of moderate physical activity five times a week. It's worth noting that these 30-minute sessions can be split into shorter intervals throughout the day to better suit your schedule.

Chair yoga is a wonderful tool to aid you in moving your joints. In a recent study by Juyoung Park (2016), Chair Yoga was investigated for its impact on osteoarthritis and was deemed a safe and effective pain management option for older adults with the condition. This leads us to our next chair yoga sequence, which emphasizes joint management.

Chair Yoga to Manage Pain

Let's look at the last ten-minute sequence we can do which will help us manage joint pain and stiffness. The suggestions for several repetitions are just that, suggestions; take more or less, whatever feels best for your body, mind, and spirit today. Similarly, adjust the size of your movements and stretches to what feels comfortable for you. Transition between poses at a pace that suits your body's needs and feels best for you in the moment.

MINDFUL AWARENESS AND CONTROLLED BREATHING

We start with this breathing technique to center ourselves and bring our breathing to a controlled even pace.

A. Take a moment to close your eyes and draw your attention inward.

B. Move your bottom forward to the front half of the chair. Rest your palms on your thighs, facing up or down, or adopt another mudra (hand position) that feels comfortable for you.

C. Plant your feet firmly at hip distance apart, your ankles right under your knees.

D. With every breath in, try to lengthen up a bit more through your spine. With every breath out, try to relax your muscles while maintaining that length.

E. After ten full breaths, or whenever you feel ready, softly blink your eyes open.

SHOULDER ROLLS TO HAND STRETCH

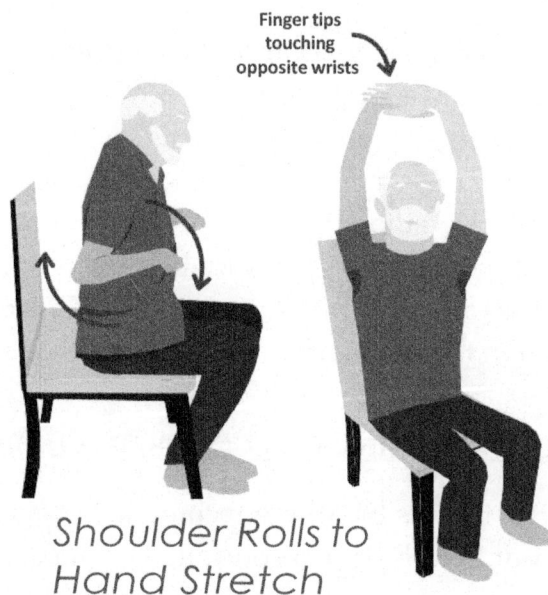

Finger tips touching opposite wrists

Shoulder Rolls to Hand Stretch

A. Seated comfortably, roll your shoulders in circles, five rotations in each direction. Do the same with your wrists.

B. Open and close your hands two times, and then give each a few good shakes.

C. Then, stretch your right arm out and upward, extending your fingers toward the sky as if signaling, "Stop!"

D. Take the left hand's palm to that right hand's palm, fingers pointing downward—so that both sets of fingertips touch the opposite hand's wrist.

E. Hold this position for five complete breaths, then shake it out. Repeat the same sequence on the other side, ending with a shake.

SEATED CAT-COW TO TORSO CIRCLES

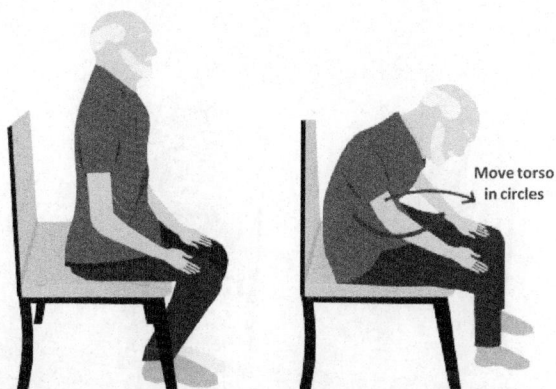

Move torso
in circles

*Seated Cat-Cow
to Torso Circles*

A. Breathe in deeply as you lift your heart towards the sky, creating a gentle arch in your back. Allow your head to follow naturally with the movement.

B. Exhale as you curve inward from your navel, making a C-shape with your spine. Allow your head to naturally follow the movement.

C. Repeat up to five times.

D. Add a side-to-side dimension to the movement by circling your torso. Complete five circles in one direction, then switch directions. Pause in stillness afterward, noticing the sensations in your body.

SEATED SUN SALUTATIONS

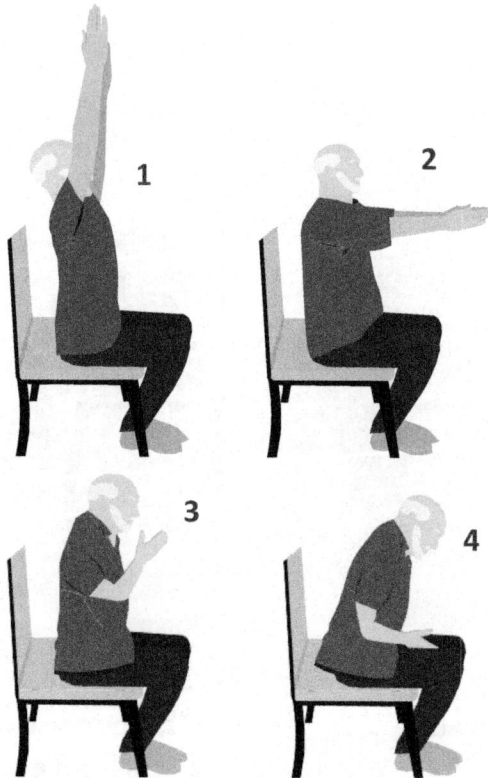

Seated Sun Salutation

A. Sitting in a chair, reach your arms out and up—or forward and up if you're in a cramped space—to meet the palms up overhead. This is *Urdhva Hastasana* (Upward Hands Pose).

B. If it's comfortable for your neck, lift your gaze to your hands, changing your perspective.

C. Reverse that movement, taking arms out and down — or through the heart center and down — to fold forward at the hips.

D. Take a full breath out, letting your head and neck release.

E. Inhale as you lift your torso slightly, and exhale as you release it fully forward again.

F. As you breathe in, lift your torso back up to the sky, extending your arms overhead to meet your palms. If it's comfortable for your neck, look up again.

G. Move your hands back through the heart center.

H. Practice up to four more rounds, you can add more as you progress in your fitness. You can add on any twists, side bends, or other movements that feel beneficial to your body.

I. Wait and breathe deeply for a few moments, allowing the sensations of movement to resonate within you.

<u>LEG CIRCLES</u>

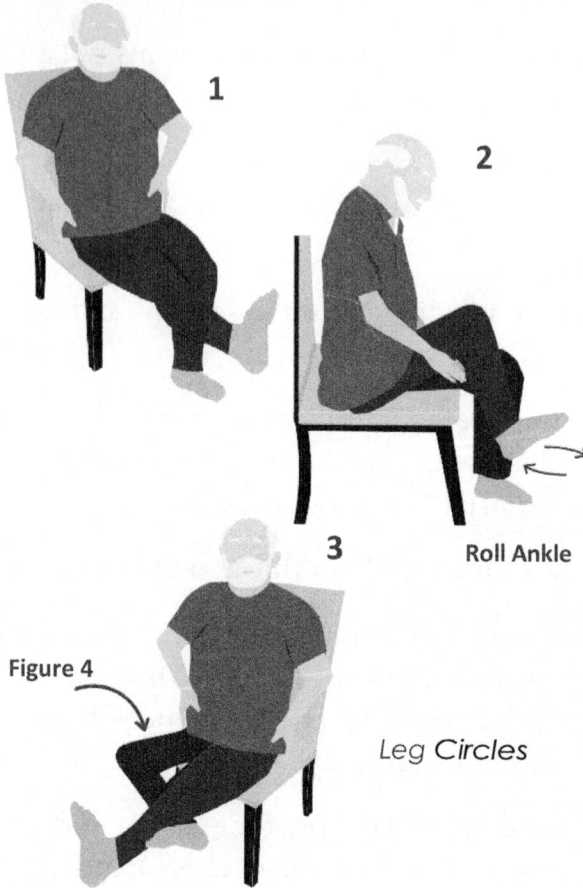

1

2

Roll Ankle

3

Figure 4

Leg *Circles*

A. Lift your right thigh a little, then extend your knee, pushing your heel forward then drop your leg back down.

B. Do the same on your left leg. Repeat four more times on each leg.

C. On the last lift, maintain your lifted thigh and reach down to clasp your hands underneath it. Then, roll the same ankle five times in each direction.

D. Then cross your ankle just above your left knee to make a "figure-4" shape. If you're not experiencing much sensation, you can use your same-side hand to apply gentle pressure to the inside of the thigh.

E. Hold for five breaths, and take the stretch on the other side.

CAMEL POSE

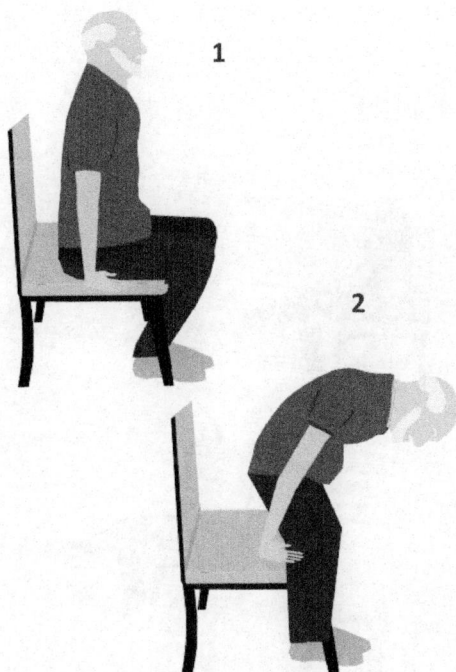

Camel Pose

A. Place your palms on the chair slightly further back from your body.

B. In a flow, from this position, inhale and raise the body, and come to your feet while holding the chair with your hands from behind.

C. Exhale when standing on your feet. Inhale, go back to sit, exhale, and come up. Repeat this three times (for six breaths).

D. While doing this, don't overstretch the abdominal muscles by throwing the chest out. Just go with the flow.

E. Release and come to relax back in the first position.

HEAD-TO-KNEE POSE

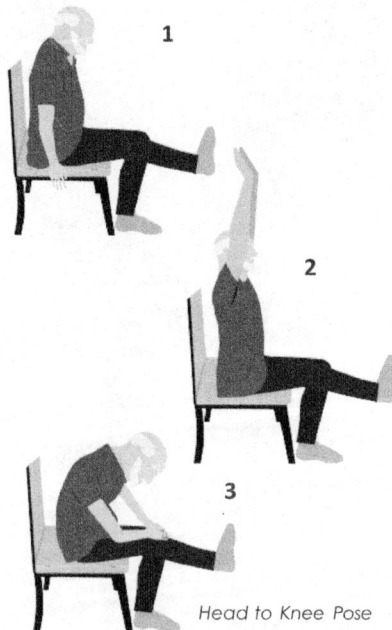

Head to Knee Pose

A. Sitting forward in your chair, straighten the right leg, toes pointing upwards, keeping the left knee bent.

B. Inhale with the arms up, as far as they will comfortably go.

C. Exhaling lean forward and keep both hands resting on the left thigh.

D. Hold for a few breaths, feeling a stretch in the right hamstring and calf.

E. Relax through the shoulders and face.

F. Try to keep the spine long. Inhaling, sit back up and change sides.

SEATED CHAIR POSE

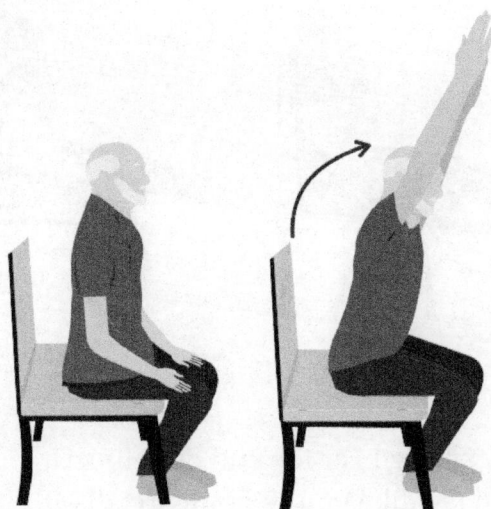

Seated Chair Pose

A. Start by sitting upright in your chair with your feet flat on the floor, and your back at a 90° angle to the floor.

B. Exhale, and lean forward so that your shoulders are about halfway across your thighs.

C. Next, inhale and raise your arms over your head with your palms facing together about shoulder-width apart.

D. Hold this pose for a few breaths.

If you want to make this pose a little easier on your lower back, don't lean as far forward.

SINGLE-LEG STRETCHES

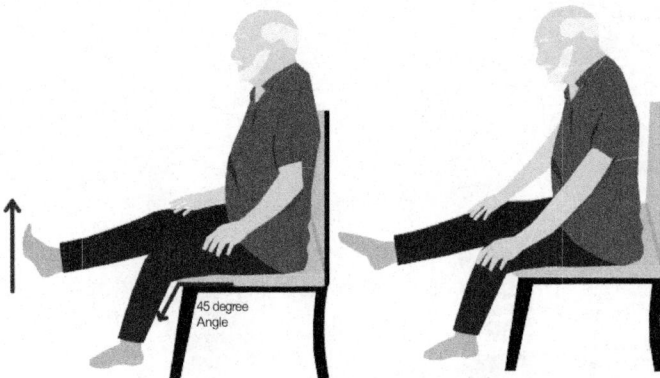

45 degree Angle

Single - Leg Stretches

A. Start by sitting near the end of your seat, but not so far that you feel like you're going to fall off.

B. Sit up straight, stretch your right leg straight, and point your right toes toward the ceiling.

C. Place your left foot flat on the floor so your left knee is bent at a 45° angle.

D. Place both hands on your leg, inhale, and make sure your spine is straight, and as you exhale, slowly slide your hands down your leg.

E. Keep your spine straight and bend at your hips, resisting the temptation to drop your head to your leg.

F. Do this for five breaths and as you breathe, slowly slide deeper into the stretch.

G. When you get out of the pose, inhale and slowly rise up, then switch sides.

CHAIR DOWNWARD DOG

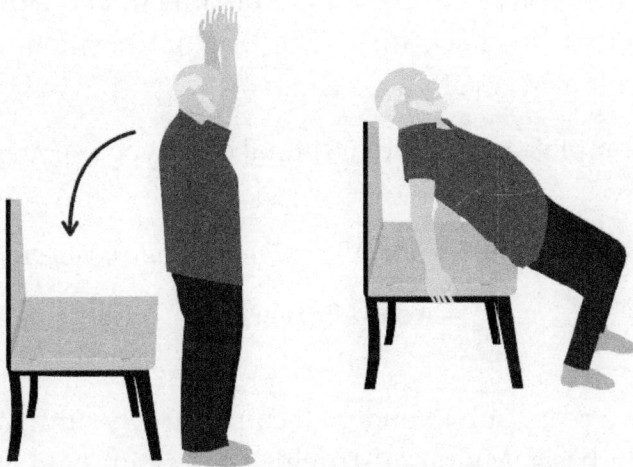

Chair Downward Dog

There are two different ways you can do this pose with a chair. You can place your hands on the seat of the chair or the top of the back of the chair. If you use the back of the chair, make sure the chair is stable enough that when you put weight on it, it doesn't move. If you do not have enough flexibility yet to place your hands on the chair, you can use a countertop or table.

A. Start by standing upright, inhaling, and lifting your hands over your head.

B. Exhale and place your hands on the back of the chair, seat, or some immovable object. Bend your knees if you need to.

C. Slowly walk your legs back so that you can feel a stretch in your shoulders, hamstrings, and calves.

D. Hold the posture for three to five breaths.

E. To get out of it, slowly walk your feet forward, and when you're close enough, breathe in and slowly lift your torso back up to the original position, raising your arms over your head.

This completes our third and final chair yoga sequence.

You can't go through life allowing pain to dictate how you behave.

— Adam Braverman

Pain is a pain, pun intended. It can destroy your happiness on a daily basis. My mom struggles with joint pain at times and finds great relief in her chair yoga practice. Her mood and social willingness improved tenfold when she managed her pain better. Medication and expert treatments are essential, especially if your doctor recommends them. However, chair yoga supplements your pain and joint health management.

Add this final sequence every third day to enjoy the benefits quickly.

CONCLUSION

With this book, our aim was to provide you with all the knowledge you need to start your journey to reclaim your health in your golden years. We have taken a look at several different aspects of health and fitness through the filter of the unique challenges that older adults tend to face when approaching this time in their lives. We understand that it is not just about the exercise, there are various aspects that go into building and regaining some of the lost fitness, strength, and mobility. This is why we took a systematic and all-round approach when introducing you to chair yoga.

First, we looked at why chair yoga could be beneficial for you. We explored what chair yoga means and some of the common misconceptions surrounding it. We also explored that when done right, it can be immensely beneficial for someone dealing with hindered mobility, fear of falling, and someone dealing with the feeling of their body not working the way their mind wants it to. We also discussed that chair yoga is not just for seniors, but anybody who might feel inclined to practice it because of certain physical issues which can restrict their ability to move.

Next, we explored preparation. It may seem simple enough but the right preparation will set you up for success. We discussed space preparations that you can do for an easy and convenient practice. As well as some things we can do to prepare our body and our mind for chair yoga. We looked at the important precautions we should take in case of certain health conditions to ensure we can practice chair yoga in a safe yet beneficial way. We talked about warm-up and cool-down sequences which we can practice before starting any chair yoga sequence to adequately prepare our system for the practice.

Further in Chapter 3, we looked at the dietary aspects which could support our practice. We discussed foods that are supportive of our systems to beat inflammation and stiffness. And also the foods which cause more inflammation and therefore should be avoided as much as possible. We also discussed some foods and dietary changes that could help us lose weight and are just generally good for our health. We end Chapter 3 with a checklist of foods that are all supportive for us and that we can include in our diet.

Chapter 4 focused more on the mind-body connection and mindfulness aspects of things. This chapter was created with the intention of providing support and resources to seniors who might be struggling with their mental health in their advanced age. Loss of confidence, increased dependence on others, the morbid reality of death, and decreased social interactions can often trigger mental health issues in older adults. Mental health is integral to our overall health and as we try to address the physical issues, we must ensure that the mental issues are also being taken care of.

We also looked at a short sleep time meditation to help you relax and get a restful sleep.

Next, we looked closely at breathwork and cardio. It might seem like an additional chore in the beginning, but adding cardio and breath-focused exercises to your routine can work wonders for your chair yoga practices. It can help you build stamina and endurance and at the same time increase your lung capacity. An increased lung capacity means your body is better oxygenated which can directly affect your energy and activity levels. Some of the cardio and breath-focused exercises can also improve your stability and balance and even improve your memory and concentration. We detailed some breathing techniques that you can practice and a short chair cardio routine to get your blood pumping.

In Chapter 6, we get into the first chair yoga routine. This sequence focuses on mobility. A lot of seniors struggle with a drop in the mobility of their limbs. We looked at why you tend to lose mobility and stability with age. We also explored some of the simple things you can do to maintain and regain your mobility and independence. Including easy stretches and low-impact cardio, essentially maintaining an active lifestyle could be a tremendous support. We looked at a ten-step, ten-minute chair yoga routine. It is a beginner-friendly routine that will help you move parts of your body that are otherwise unused.

The next chapter focuses on strength. We tend to rapidly lose muscle mass as we age. this causes a drop in strength and increases frailty among seniors. We discussed sarcopenia in detail, the loss of muscle fiber, and how both of these things can affect our lives as we age. The good news is that muscles can be gained back to a great extent if we just train right and eat right. Eating protein-rich food is key to gaining your muscle strength back along with exercises, preferably resistance training. Improving your muscle strength and power can also help improve your reflexes and protect you from injuries. We detailed our second chair yoga sequence next where the focus is on improving your strength.

Our last chapter is all about joint health. Joint pain and degeneration is another huge issue faced by the older population. In this chapter, we took a closer look at why it is so and how certain chronic conditions can affect joint health. We also explored the behavioral changes we can make to support our joints like losing weight and getting better sleep. We examined the role of supplements in improving our joint health as well. We end with a chair yoga sequence which focuses on joint mobility and strength. This is also a beginner-friendly sequence and aims to provide easy-to-follow yet effective exercises.

My mother is still going strong, and we love her quirky influence over our lives. She is such a blessing and is a key part of our family. We keep her active as much as she feels comfortable. After all, she is 89. Sometimes, she loves spending the day at home watching her favorite gameshows or playing a game with one of her friends. Her mental habits have truly strengthened her as she gained the strength to reduce the risk of falling and remain as mobile as she wished and when she wished. That's one of the secrets she wanted me to share. My mom suggests you work on strengthening your muscles, managing your mobility, and sustaining independence as long as it fits your comfort levels.

But don't push yourself overboard as there comes a point when taking it easy matters, as well. Instead, enjoy resting and solving puzzles with family and friends. Enjoy dinner with loved ones and tell them all about your amazing stories. The salvation that comes with aging is nostalgia and the joy of sharing it.

Be as active as you can and wish to be. Don't stop your chair yoga, breathwork, and light cardio, they help you stay healthy. My mother, my family, and I all wish you the best and hope you enjoy the asanas! We'd love to know how these chair yoga workout sequences helped you. If it has, please leave a favorable review on Amazon, which will help others find this information. Lastly, embrace your golden years with everything you already have and will gain through this daily practice. Blessings.

~ Roman

GLOSSARY

- **Achilles Tendon:** the strong tendon connecting the calf muscles to the bone of the heel.

- **Adrenaline:** the hormone triggering the body's fight-or-flight reaction to stress, occurs during hazardous, alarming, or intensely competitive circumstances.

- **Alveolar Dead Space:** the alveoli that receive air from outside but are not connected to the arteries to exchange carbon dioxide with oxygen.

- **Alzheimer's:** a degenerative brain disorder, represents the predominant type of dementia. It commonly starts in late middle age or old age, resulting in progressive memory decline, confusion, cognitive impairment, and alterations in personality and mood.

- **Antioxidants:** a substance that inhibits reactions promoted by oxygen, peroxides, or free radicals.

- **Anxiety:** an abnormal sense of stress, apprehension, or fear often marked by physical signs.

- **Apoptosis:** an abnormal and overwhelming sense of apprehension and fear often marked by physical signs.

- **Arterial Oxygen:** oxygen in the arteries.

175

- **Ashtanga Yoga:** Ashtanga yoga is a dynamic style of classical Indian yoga.

- **Autoimmune Disease:** a disease caused when the defensive cells of the body start attacking molecules, cells, or tissues of the body itself.

- **Breathwork:** conscious, controlled breathing with a focus on relaxation and meditation.

- **Bursitis:** inflammation of a bursa, such as those found in the shoulder or elbow.

- **Buteyko Breathing:** entails a complementary or alternative physical therapy, advocating breathing exercises primarily for conditions like asthma and an unspecified degenerative brain disease, which is the prevalent form of dementia.

- **C- Reactive Protein:** a protein produced in the liver and normally found in blood plasma. Its levels in circulation increase in response to inflammation.

- **Carpal Tunnel Syndrome:** develops due to the compression of a nerve as it passes through the wrist into the hand. This compression leads to weakness, sensory disturbances, and discomfort in the hand and fingers.

- **Chair Yoga:** a form of yoga that involves doing yoga sequences while sitting on a chair or using the chair for support.

- **Cholesterol:** a fat-like compound characterized by its waxy consistency, distributed throughout the cells, tissues, and bodily fluids of humans and animals.

- **Chronic Conditions:** a disease that continues or occurs again and again for a long time: a medical condition of prolonged duration.

- **Chronic Fatigue Syndrome:** a disorder that is characterized by persistent fatigue.

- **Chronic Inflammation:** It occurs when there is an injury or a foreign body and the inflammatory cells travel there in response to this external injury or event. If inflammatory cells stay too long, it is called chronic inflammation.

- **Cognitive Behavioral Therapy:** psychotherapy that involves identifying patterns of thinking, behavior, or emotions and substituting them with desirable ways of doing the same.

- **Collagen:** a group of fibrous proteins prevalent in vertebrates, acting as the principal component within connective tissue fibrils and bones.

- **Cortisol:** a glucocorticoid produced by the adrenal cortex when stimulated by ACTH. It facilitates numerous metabolic functions, such as gluconeogenesis, possesses anti-inflammatory and immunosuppressive attributes, and its blood levels may become elevated in reaction to physical or psychological stress.

- **Crohn's Disease:** a chronic inflammatory condition primarily affecting the lower part of the ileum, with frequent extension into the colon. It presents symptoms such as diarrhea, abdominal cramping, reduced appetite, weight loss, and the formation of abscesses and scar tissue.

- **Cytokines:** a category of immunoregulatory proteins, such as interleukin or interferon, which are nearby cells, predominantly those of the immune system.

- **Dementia:** a condition that causes cognitive deficits and is usually progressive in nature.

- **Depression:** a state of feeling sad and having a depressive mood for long periods of time.

- **Diabetes:** any abnormal condition where there is an imbalance of insulin in the body.

- **Diaphragmatic Breathing:** a deep breathing exercise that engages the diaphragm.

- **Estradiol:** a natural estrogenic hormone that is secreted chiefly by the ovaries, and that is used to treat menopausal symptoms.

- **Estrogen:** any of various natural steroids (such as estradiol) that are secreted chiefly by the female reproductive system for growth and maintenance.

- **Foot Flexion:** a movement in which the top of your foot points away from your leg.

- **Glucosamine:** an amino derivative of glucose, primarily found as a component of various polysaccharides forming structural substances.

- • **Gout:** a metabolic disease characterized by painful joint inflammation and the accumulation of urates in and around the joints.

- **Hatha Yoga:** a practice of physical exercises for mastering and refining the body, forming an integral part of the four principal Hindu disciplines.

- **Hyaluronic Acid:** a viscous fluid that serves as a structural element and lubricant.

- **Hypertension:** is characterized by unusually high blood pressure, especially arterial blood pressure.

- **Immune Response:** a response that occurs when the body identifies a molecule as foreign and induces the formation of antibodies to counter it.

- **Insulin Resistance:** is characterized by reduced sensitivity to insulin in the body's insulin-dependent processes, normally observed in type 2 diabetes but can occur even without diabetes.

- **Intercostal Muscles:** muscles situated or extending between the ribs.

- **Intermittent Fasting:** involves alternating between periods of eating and fasting as an eating pattern.

- **Lipids:** substances that are not water soluble and form structural components of living cells.

- **Lupus:** any of several diseases characterized by skin lesions.

- **Menopause:** is the natural cessation of menstruation that typically occurs between the ages of 45 and 55.

- **Metabolic Syndrome:** refers to a syndrome marked by the presence of usually three or more factors that are associated with a increased risk of cardiovascular disease and type 2 diabetes.

- **Mindfulness:** the practice of maintaining a state of heightened awareness of one's thoughts, experiences, and emotions.

- **Mitochondrial:** are cellular organelles found in most eukaryotes, existing outside the nucleus. They produce energy for the cell through cellular respiration and are rich in fats, proteins, and enzymes.

- **Muscular Dystrophy:** refers to a group of hereditary diseases marked by progressive muscle wasting.

- **Multiple Sclerosis:** is a disease marked by patches of hardened tissue in the brain or spinal cord, often linked with partial or complete paralysis and jerking muscle tremors.

- **Osteoarthritis:** a common form of arthritis that is marked by stiffness, pain, swelling, and deformation of joints because of degenerative changes in the cartilage.

- **Osteopenia:** a reduction in bone volume below normal levels, often resulting from insufficient replacement of bone lost through regular breakdown (lysis).

- **Osteoporosis:** a condition featuring a decline in bone mass with decreased density, and the expansion of bone spaces, ultimately rendering the bones weak and prone to fragility.

- **Panic Attacks:** are brief episodes of intense fear or dread, abruptly appearing and typically diminishing within 30 minutes. They usually occur without a clear cause but may occasionally be linked to a recognizable triggering stimulus.

- **Parathyroid:** of, relating to, or produced by the parathyroid glands.

- **Polycystic Ovarian Syndrome:** a variable disease where there is an imbalance of the sex hormones and that is marked by amenorrhea, hirsutism, obesity, infertility, and ovarian enlargement.

- **Power Yoga:** a blend of yoga styles emphasizing the building of strength and endurance.

- **Pranayama:** yogic breath control or a technique used in yogic breath control.

- **Prediabetes:** a state that precedes the development of diabetes.

- **Psoriatic Arthritis:** a severe arthritis variant distinguished by joint inflammation, concurrent psoriasis affecting the skin or nails, and a negative test for rheumatoid factor.

- **Rehabilitation:** restoration of physical function by therapeutic means.

- **Rheumatoid Arthritis:** is typically a chronic autoimmune condition known for pain, stiffness, inflammation, swelling, and sometimes joint destruction.

- **Sarcopenia:** reduction in skeletal muscle mass due to aging.

- **Spine Flexion:** the act of bending forward.

- **Spine Rotation:** the act of twisting toward the back.

- **Synovial Fluid:** a transparent lubricating fluid found in between the joints.

- **Tendinitis:** inflammation of a tendon, often linked with acute injury, and normally accompanied by pain and swelling.

- **Testosterone:** a hormone produced by the testes, playing a key role in the development and maintenance of male secondary sex characteristics.

- **Thoracic Cavity:** the cavity of the thorax that is just above the diaphragm, and is enclosed by the sternum, ribs, and vertebrae on all the other sides. It contains the heart and lungs.

- **Type 2 Diabetes:** a common form of diabetes marked by increased blood sugar levels due to impaired insulin utilization, coupled with the body's inability to adequately increase insulin production.

- **Ulcerative Colitis:** an inflammatory disease of the colon that is not clearly understood. It presents with symptoms such as diarrhea accompanied by mucus and blood, abdominal pain with cramps, and inflammation and swelling of the mucous membrane, featuring ulcerated patches.

- **Vinyasa Yoga:** a style of yoga where you move from one to another, seamlessly, using breath in a way that supports the smooth movements.

- **Yogasana:** The practice of yoga postures or yoga poses.

References

5 Best Meditation Podcasts for Seniors. (2016, May 16). Lifetime Daily. https://www.lifetimedaily.com/5-best-meditation-podcasts-for-seniors

8 Foods Older Adults Should Avoid Eating. (2016, November 29). Sun Health Communities. https://www.sunhealthcommunities.org/helpful-tools/articles/8-foods-older-adults-avoid-eating

8 Yoga Myths to Stop Believing Today. (2019, June 21). Cleveland Clinic. https://health.clevelandclinic.org/think-you-cant-do-yoga-you-might-be-believing-one-of-these-8-yoga-myths

15 inspirational quotes about aging and lifelong learning. (2021, March 15). Tea and Toast. https://www.teaandtoast.ca/blog/15-quotes-aging-learning

6 Ways to Maintain Mobility as You Age Five Star Senior Living. (2020, March 6). Five Star Senior Living. https://www.fivestarseniorliving.com/blog/6-ways-to-maintain-mobility-as-you-age-amalateesside. (2022, January 5). *Sarcopenia - 8 ways how Chair Based Yoga and Exercise can help fight muscle loss as we age.*

AMALAwellness.
https://amalateesside.com/2022/01/05/sarcopenia-8-
ways-how-chair-based-yoga-and-exercise-can-help-fight-
muscle-loss-as-we-age

American Lung Association. (2019). *Lung Capacity and Aging*.
https://www.lung.org/lung-health-diseases/how-lungs-
work/lung-capacity-and-aging

Bastin, A. (2021, August 13). *The Benefits of Low-Impact
Workout Routines for Older Adults*. Lifeline.
https://www.lifeline.com/blog/low-impact-exercise-for-
senior-health-and-happiness/

Better Health Channel. (2015). *Ageing - muscles bones and
joints*.
https://www.betterhealth.vic.gov.au/health/conditionsa
ndtreatments/ageing-muscles-bones-and-joints

Brandy, B. (2021, August 16). *Natural Anti-Inflammatory Foods
Seniors Should Be Eating*. Rittenhouse Village.
https://www.rittenhousevillages.com/assisted-living-
blog/natural-anti-inflammatory-foods-seniors-should-be-
eating

Brown, M. J. (2017, June 15). *Fresh vs Frozen Fruit and
Vegetables — Which Are Healthier?* Healthline.
https://www.healthline.com/nutrition/fresh-vs-frozen-
fruit-and-vegetables#TOC_TITLE_HDR_3

Carelink Staff. (2021, April 27). *How to Maintain Mobility in
Old Age*. CareLink. https://www.carelink.org/how-to-
maintain-mobility-in-old-age/

Centers for Disease Control and Prevention. (2019). *How
much physical activity do older adults need?*

https://www.cdc.gov/physicalactivity/basics/older_ad
ults/index.htm

Chair Exercises for Seniors. (n.d.). Senior Services of America.
https://seniorservicesofamerica.com/blog/chair-
exercises-for-seniors/

Chair Flexing Foot Pose Yoga. (2018, July 26). Tummee.com.
https://www.tummee.com/yoga-poses/chair-flexing-
foot-pose

Chair Neck Rolls B Yoga. (2017, October 15). Tummee.com.
https://www.tummee.com/yoga-poses/chair-neck-rolls-
b

Chair Seated Warm Up Flow Yoga. (n.d.). Tummee.com.
https://www.tummee.com/yoga-poses/chair-seated-
warm-up-flow

Chair Yoga for Seniors: 7 Poses To Support Mobility. (2020,
August 14). Snug Safety. https://www.snugsafe.com/all-
posts/chair-yoga-for-seniors

Chair Yoga Poses | How to get started with chair yoga. (n.d.).
University of Arkansas System.
https://www.uaex.uada.edu/life-skills-
wellness/health/physical-activity-resources/chair-
yoga.aspx

Cleveland Clinic. (2022, June 3). *Sarcopenia (Muscle Loss):
Symptoms & Causes.*
https://my.clevelandclinic.org/health/diseases/23167-
sarcopenia

Cristol, H. (2019, October 30). *Rheumatoid Arthritis vs.
Osteoarthritis: What's the Difference?* WebMD.

https://www.webmd.com/rheumatoid-arthritis/rheumatoid-arthritis-osteoarthritis-difference

Culinary Services Group. (2020, August 5). *Anti-Inflammatory Diets and Menus for Seniors.* https://culinaryservicesgroup.com/anti-inflammatory-menus-for-seniors

Davis, J. L. (2003, February 3). *Joint Pain Not Inevitable With Age.* WebMD; WebMD. https://www.webmd.com/osteoarthritis/features/joint-pain-management-age

DeCataldo, J. (2023, January 1). *Chair Yoga and Why Seated Yoga Poses Are Good For You.* Lifespan. https://www.lifespan.org/lifespan-living/chair-yoga-and-why-seated-yoga-poses-are-good-you

Drake, K. (2022, June 22). *What Is Chair Yoga? What Are Its Benefits?* GoodRx. https://www.goodrx.com/well-being/movement-exercise/chair-yoga

Ferrucci, L., & Fabbri, E. (2018). Inflammageing: chronic inflammation in ageing, cardiovascular disease, and frailty. *Nature Reviews Cardiology, 15*(9), 505–522. https://doi.org/10.1038/s41569-018-0064-2

Fiorenzi, R. (2019, July 23). *Best Chair Yoga Poses for Back Pain.* Start Standing. https://www.startstanding.org/sitting-back-pain/best-chair-yoga-poses-for-back-pain

Fischer, A. (2023, February 22). *Here's What to Add to Your Grocery List if You're Trying to Lose Weight.* Good Housekeeping. https://www.goodhousekeeping.com/health/diet-nutrition/a42747909/weight-loss-grocery-list/

Foods that Cause Inflammation. (2020, March 30). Savory Living. https://www.savoryliving.com/foods-that-cause-inflammation

Freemont, A., & Hoyland, J. (2007). Morphology, mechanisms and pathology of musculoskeletal ageing. *The Journal of Pathology, 211*(2), 252–259. https://doi.org/10.1002/path.2097

Galantino, M., DeCesari, J., Rinaldi, S., Wurst, V., Nell, M., Green, L., MacKain, N., Stevens, M., Marsico, R., & Mao, J. (2012). Safety and feasibility of modified chair-yoga on functional outcome among elderly at risk for falls. *International Journal of Yoga, 5*(2), 146. https://doi.org/10.4103/0973-6131.98242

Geraci, A., Calvani, R., Ferri, E., Marzetti, E., Arosio, B., & Cesari, M. (2021). Sarcopenia and Menopause: The Role of Estradiol. *Frontiers in Endocrinology, 12.* https://doi.org/10.3389/fendo.2021.682012

Good Man Group. (n.d.). *6 Mindfulness Activities for Senior Wellness.* https://blog.thegoodmangroup.com/mindfulness-activities-for-seniors

Grebeniuk, N. M., I. (2022, August 16). *Chair Yoga For Seniors: 10 Poses To Improve Strength, Flexibility, And Balance.* BetterMe Blog. https://betterme.world/articles/chair-yoga-for-seniors

Hart, P. (2019). *What Is the Mind-Body Connection?* Taking Charge of Your Health & Wellbeing. https://www.takingcharge.csh.umn.edu/what-is-the-mind-body-connection

Harvard Health Publishing. (2016, February 19). *Preserve your muscle mass.* Harvard Health. https://www.health.harvard.edu/staying-healthy/preserve-your-muscle-mass

Harvard Health Publishing. (2021, January 2). *Protecting against cognitive decline.* Harvard Health. https://www.health.harvard.edu/mind-and-mood/protecting-against-cognitive-decline

Hellicar, L. (2022, September 16). *What Is yogic breathing? Benefits, types, and how to try.* Medicalnews Today. https://www.medicalnewstoday.com/articles/what-is-yogic-breathing

Home Instead. (2022, January 14). *10 Quotes About the Beauty of Aging.* https://www.homeinstead.com/location/529/news-and-media/10-quotes-about-the-beauty-of-aging

How to Choose a Chair for Yoga. (2014, May 4). Yoga with Grace. https://www.yogawithgrace.net/pams-blog/how-to-choose-a-chair-for-yoga

How to teach Chair Yoga Head To Knee Pose (Janu Sirasana). (n.d.). GeorgeWatts.org. https://georgewatts.org/lesson-planner/yoga_pilates_poses/chair-yoga-head-to-knee-janu-sirasana/

Hughes, L. (2022, November 28). *How To Teach Chair Yoga: Step-By-Step Guide.* Origym Personal Trainer Courses. https://origympersonaltrainercourses.co.uk/blog/teaching-chair-yoga

Joint Pain: Symptoms, Causes, and Treatment. (2018, March 28). Cleveland Clinic.

https://my.clevelandclinic.org/health/symptoms/17752-joint-pain

Kendal at Home. (2023, September 13). *Eight (8) Simple Breathing Exercises for Older Adults.* https://www.kendalathome.org/blog/breathe-easy-six-breath-exercises-for-older-adults

Kertapati, Y., Sahar, J., & Nursasi, A. Y. (2018). The effects of chair yoga with spiritual intervention on the functional status of older adults. *Enfermeria Clinica, 28 Suppl 1*, 70–73. https://doi.org/10.1016/S1130-8621(18)30040-8

Kubala, J. (2019, May 13). *The 20 Best Ways to Lose Weight After 50.* Healthline. https://www.healthline.com/nutrition/how-to-lose-weight-after-50

Kujala, U. M., Hautasaari, P., Vähä-Ypyä, H., Waller, K., Lindgren, N., Iso-Markku, P., Heikkilä, K., Rinne, J., Kaprio, J., & Sievänen, H. (2019). Chronic diseases and objectively monitored physical activity profile among aged individuals – a cross-sectional twin cohort study. *Annals of Medicine, 51*(1), 78–87. https://doi.org/10.1080/07853890.2019.1566765

Landry, J., BS, & RRT. (2023, March 23). *99+ Best Quotes About Breathing (Respiratory Edition).* Respiratory Therapy Zone. https://www.respiratorytherapyzone.com/quotes-about-breathing

Linda. (2021, February 3). *Anti-Inflammatory Foods Seniors Should Add to Their Diet.* AZNHA. https://aznha.org/anti-inflammatory-foods-seniors-should-add-to-their-diet-2

Lutz, J. (2018, July 10). *Chair Yoga: Gentle, Effective Exercise for Osteoarthritis Pain*. Health Central. https://www.healthcentral.com/condition/osteoarthritis /chair-yoga-gentle-effective-exercise-osteoarthritis-pain

Maintaining Mobility As Part Of Healthy Aging. (2010). Nestle Health Science. https://www.nestlehealthscience.com/health-management/aging/maintaining-mobility-as-part-of-healthy-aging

Mayo Clinic Staff. (2020, September 15). *Mindfulness exercises*. Mayo Clinic. https://www.mayoclinic.org/healthy-lifestyle/consumer-health/in-depth/mindfulness-exercises/art-20046356

Megala, J. (2022, January 20). *Why Your Mobility Worsens As You Age, and What to Do About It*. Livestrong. https://www.livestrong.com/article/13768998-loss-of-mobility-aging/

Menezes, L. (2020, August 24). *What is the Mind-Body Connection?* Florida Medical Clinic. https://www.floridamedicalclinic.com/blog/what-is-the-mind-body-connection

Messier, S. P., Gutekunst, D. J., Davis, C., & DeVita, P. (2005). Weight loss reduces knee-joint loads in overweight and obese older adults with knee osteoarthritis. *Arthritis & Rheumatism, 52*(7), 2026–2032. https://doi.org/10.1002/art.21139

Mind Over Body Quotes (4 quotes). (n.d.). Goodreads. https://www.goodreads.com/quotes/tag/mind-over-body

Mitchell, C. (2014, September 4). *Seniors and Mental Health.* Pan American Health Organization / World Health Organization. https://www3.paho.org/hq/index.php?option=com_con tent&view=article&id=9877:seniors-mental- health&Itemid=0&lang=en

Moniuszko, S. M. (2022, March 23). *"Glimmers" are the opposite of triggers. Here's how to embrace them.* USA TODAY. https://www.usatoday.com/story/life/health- wellness/2022/03/23/glimmers-opposite-triggers- mental-health-benefits/7121353001/

National Institute on Aging. (2020, April 3). *How older adults can get started with exercise.* https://www.nia.nih.gov/health/how-older-adults-can- get-started-exercise

National Institute on Aging. (2022, September 12). *Older Adults and Balance Problems.* https://www.nia.nih.gov/health/older-adults-and- balance-problems

National Institutes of Health. (2021, June 1). *Mindfulness for your health.* NIH News in Health. https://newsinhealth.nih.gov/2021/06/mindfulness- your-health

Nour, M., Lutze, S., Grech, A., & Allman-Farinelli, M. (2018). The Relationship between Vegetable Intake and Weight Outcomes: A Systematic Review of Cohort Studies. *Nutrients, 10*(11), 1626. https://doi.org/10.3390/nu10111626

Osmanski, S. (2023, June 13). *50 Chronic Pain Quotes To Inspire*. Parade. https://parade.com/1185268/stephanieosmanski/chroni c-pain-quotes

Pain Doctor. (2019, September 16). *Chair Yoga For Seniors And Those With Limited Mobility: 12 Poses To Try*. Pain Doctor. https://paindoctor.com/chair-yoga-for-seniors/

Park, J., McCaffrey, R., Newman, D., Cheung, C., & Hagen, D. (2014). The Effect of Sit "N" Fit Chair Yoga Among Community-Dwelling Older Adults With Osteoarthritis. *Holistic Nursing Practice, 28*(4), 247. https://www.academia.edu/81033246/The_Effect_of_Sit _N_Fit_Chair_Yoga_Among_Community_Dwelling_Olde r_Adults_With_Osteoarthritis

Park, J., McCaffrey, R., Newman, D., Liehr, P., & Ouslander, J. G. (2016). A Pilot Randomized Controlled Trial of the Effects of Chair Yoga on Pain and Physical Function Among Community-Dwelling Older Adults With Lower Extremity Osteoarthritis. *Journal of the American Geriatrics Society, 65*(3), 592–597. https://doi.org/10.1111/jgs.14717

Park, J., Tolea, M. I., Sherman, D., Rosenfeld, A., Arcay, V., Lopes, Y., & Galvin, J. E. (2020). Feasibility of Conducting Nonpharmacological Interventions to Manage Dementia Symptoms in Community-Dwelling Older Adults: A Cluster Randomized Controlled Trial. *American Journal of Alzheimer's Disease and Other Dementias, 35*, 1533317519872635. https://doi.org/10.1177/1533317519872635

Passalacqua, B. (2023, March 16). *Yoga Therapy for Muscular Dystrophy: Benefits, How to, and More.* Breathing Deeply. https://breathingdeeply.com/yt-muscular-dystrophy

Perkins, T. (2023, February 8). *Chair Yoga Myths.* Trin Perkins. https://trinperkins.com/chair-yoga-myths

Physical activity guidelines for older adults. (2022, January 25). Nhs.uk. https://www.nhs.uk/live-well/exercise/exercise-guidelines/physical-activity-guidelines-older-adults

Physiopedia. (2019a). *Effects of Ageing on Joints.* https://www.physio-pedia.com/Effects_of_Ageing_on_Joints

Physiopedia. (2019b). *Muscle Function: Effects of Aging.* https://www.physio-pedia.com/Muscle_Function:_effects_of_aging

pmjiii. (2022, November 3). *Chair Yoga Precautions.* Aura Wellness Center. https://aurawellnesscenter.com/2022/11/03/chair-yoga-precautions

Public Relations Staff. (2023). *APA report: Lack of willpower may be obstacle to improving personal health and finances.* APA Services. https://www.apaservices.org/practice/update/2012/02-23/willpower

Ramirez, D. (n.d.). *Breath Awareness.* Positive Psychology. https://positive.b-cdn.net/wp-content/uploads/Breath-Awareness.pdf

Rashmi, S. M., & Ames, D. (2016). Impact of a 10 minute Seated Yoga Practice in the Management of Diabetes. *Journal of Yoga & Physical Therapy*, *06*(01). https://doi.org/10.4172/2157-7595.1000224

Ross, S. A., Domínguez, S., Nigam, N., & Wakeling, J. M. (2021). The Energy of Muscle Contraction. III. Kinetic Energy During Cyclic Contractions. *Frontiers in Physiology*, *12*. https://doi.org/10.3389/fphys.2021.628819

Rucki, J. A. (2022, June 1). *Chair yoga*. Buffalo Spree. https://www.buffalospree.com/style_living/healthy_life styles/chair-yoga/article_4bfde06e-dd1e-11ec-a298-0fb3e1e3bd81.html

Senior Lifestyle. (2020a, February 4). 7 Best Exercises for Seniors (and a Few to Avoid!). https://www.seniorlifestyle.com/resources/blog/7-best-exercises-for-seniors-and-a-few-to-avoid

Senior Lifestyle. (2020b, February 12). Top 10 Chair Yoga Positions for Seniors [Infographic]. https://www.seniorlifestyle.com/resources/blog/infogr aphic-top-10-chair-yoga-positions-for-seniors

Schmid, A. A., van Puymbroeck, M., & Koceja, D. M. (2010). Effect of a 12-Week Yoga Intervention on Fear of Falling and Balance in Older Adults: A Pilot Study. *Archives of Physical Medicine and Rehabilitation*, *91*(4), 576–583. https://doi.org/10.1016/j.apmr.2009.12.018

Schulz, C. (2020, May 4). *Mobility Quotes - 39 Sayings for the Sustainable Locomotion of the Future*. CareElite. https://www.careelite.de/en/sustainable-mobility-quotes

Selhub, E. (2022, September 18). *Nutritional psychiatry: Your brain on food*. Harvard Health Publishing. https://www.health.harvard.edu/blog/nutritional-psychiatry-your-brain-on-food-201511168626

Sherrel, Z. (2022, November 23). *All my joints hurt suddenly: 10 causes and their treatment*. Medical News Today. https://www.medicalnewstoday.com/articles/all-my-joints-hurt-suddenly

Shifu Shirley Chock, CCWS. (n.d.). Aiping Tai Chi Center. https://aipingtaichi.com/shifu-shirley-chock/

Silver Cuisine Team. (2017, June 20). *10 Foods to Avoid After 60*. Silver Cuisine. https://blog.silvercuisine.com/8-foods-seniors-should-never-eat

Sitting exercises. (2022, January 26). Nhs.uk. https://www.nhs.uk/live-well/exercise/strength-and-flexibility-exercises/sitting-exercises

Smith, E. N. (2019, June 1). *A Chair Yoga Sequence for Arthritis: Increase Mobility and Decrease Pain*. YogaUOnline. https://yogauonline.com/yoga-and-healthy-aging/yoga-for-arthritis/a-chair-yoga-sequence-for-arthritis-increase-mobility-and-decrease-pain

Smith, S. (2020, June 29). *3 Misconceptions and 3 Fun Facts About Chair Yoga*. Rise + Vibe. https://www.riseandvibeyoga.com/blog/chair-yoga

Stein, N. (2018, March 4). *10 Surprising Foods with Added Sugars*. Lark.com. https://www.lark.com/resources/10-surprising-foods-with-added-sugars

Stumm, B. (2022, September 21). *Meditation Resources for Seniors: Useful Tips and Tricks.* Brettstumm.com. https://brettstumm.com/best-meditation-resource-for-seniors

Supported Chair Camel Pose Yoga (Salamba Chair Ustrasana). (2018, July 27). Tummee.com. https://www.tummee.com/yoga-poses/supported-chair-camel-pose

Swenson, P. D., & Kaplan, M. H. (1987). Comparison of two rapid culture methods for detection of cytomegalovirus in clinical specimens. *Journal of Clinical Microbiology, 25*(12), 2445–2446. https://www.ncbi.nlm.nih.gov/pmc/articles/PMC269517

The Effects of Depression in Your Body. (2022, September 21). Healthline. https://www.healthline.com/health/depression/effects-on-body#fa-qs

The effects of depression on the body and physical health. (n.d.). Medical News Today. https://www.medicalnewstoday.com/articles/322395#outlook

The Mindfulness Meditation Techniques. (n.d.). Mindfulness Meditation Institute. https://mindfulnessmeditationinstitute.org/the-mindfulness-meditation-practice/mindfulness-meditation-techniques

tjeffries. (2022, November 19). *13 Chair Yoga Poses for Seniors.* Yoga Journal.

https://www.yogajournal.com/practice/chair-yoga-for-seniors/

Upper Hand. (2021, April 25). *Top 50 Motivational Workout Quotes*. https://upperhand.com/50-motivational-workout-quotes

Vive Health. (2018, October 6). *50 Cardio Exercises for Seniors*. https://www.vivehealth.com/blogs/resources/cardio-exercises-for-seniors

Wallace, R. (2015, April 14). *The Link Between Weight Loss and Knee Pain*. Healthline. https://www.healthline.com/health/osteoarthritis/knee-pain/link-between-weight-loss-and-knee-pain

WebMD Editorial Contributors. (2021, June 28). *What Is Breathwork?* WebMD. https://www.webmd.com/balance/what-is-breathwork

What Chair is Good for Chair Yoga? (2021, February 9). Flowithme. https://www.flowithme.com/post/what-chair-is-good-for-chair-yoga

What to Know About Breathing When Running. (2023, July 21). WebMD. https://www.webmd.com/fitness-exercise/what-to-know-breathing-when-running

Yao, C.-T., Lee, B.-O., Hong, H., & Su, Y.-C. (2023). Effect of Chair Yoga Therapy on Functional Fitness and Daily Life Activities among Older Female Adults with Knee Osteoarthritis in Taiwan: A Quasi-Experimental Study. *Healthcare, 11*(7), 1024. https://doi.org/10.3390/healthcare11071024

Yoga for Seniors: Benefits, Poses, Chair Yoga. (n.d.). Lifeline. https://www.lifeline.ca/en/resources/yoga-for-senior

You Are What You Eat Quotes (11 quotes). (n.d.). Goodreads. https://www.goodreads.com/quotes/tag/you-are-what-you-eat

Yu, Z. M., DeClercq, V., Cui, Y., Forbes, C., Grandy, S., Keats, M., Parker, L., Sweeney, E., & Dummer, T. J. B. (2018). Fruit and vegetable intake and body adiposity among populations in Eastern Canada: the Atlantic Partnership for Tomorrow's Health Study. *BMJ Open,* *8*(4), e018060. https://doi.org/10.1136/bmjopen-2017-018060

Yuan, X., Wang, J., Yang, S., Gao, M., Cao, L., Li, X., Hong, D., Tian, S., & Sun, C. (2022). Effect of Intermittent Fasting Diet on Glucose and Lipid Metabolism and Insulin Resistance in Patients with Impaired Glucose and Lipid Metabolism: A Systematic Review and Meta-Analysis. *International Journal of Endocrinology, 2022,* 1–9. https://doi.org/10.1155/2022/6999907

Zheng, G., Li, S., Huang, M., Liu, F., Tao, J., & Chen, L. (2015). The Effect of Tai Chi Training on Cardiorespiratory Fitness in Healthy Adults: A Systematic Review and Meta-Analysis. *PLOS ONE, 10*(2), e0117360. https://doi.org/10.1371/journal.pone.0117360

Image References

Aurelius, M. (2021). *healthy-woman-relaxation-garden* [Image]. Pexels. https://www.pexels.com/photo/healthy-woman-relaxation-garden-6787202/

Bijutoha. (2019, June 18). *chair-chair-png-transparent-image* [Image]. Pixabay. https://pixabay.com/illustrations/chair-chair-png-transparent-image-4281511/

cottonbro studio. (2020, July 23). *blonde-woman-in-black-skirt-and-white-dress-shirt-walking-her-dalmatian-dog* [Image]. Pexels. https://www.pexels.com/photo/blonde-woman-in-black-skirt-and-white-dress-shirt-walking-her-dalmatian-dog-4936456/

energepic.com. (2017, February 3). *woman-sitting-in-front-of-macbook* [Image]. Pexels. https://www.pexels.com/photo/woman-sitting-in-front-of-macbook-313690/

Flat Lay Photography. (2018, August 28). *Assorted Variety of stir fried and vegetable foods* [Image]. Unsplash.com. https://unsplash.com/photos/flat-lay-photography-of-assorted-variety-of-stir-fried-and-vegetable-foods-3iexvMShGfQ

Hayley Lawrence. (2019, December 16). *White Metal Folding Chair* [Image]. Unsplash.com. https://unsplash.com/photos/white-metal-folding-chair-ddVgLbbS66o

Iograstudio. (2019, April 15). *woman-stretch-fitness-outdoor* [Image]. Pixabay. https://pixabay.com/photos/woman-stretch-fitness-outdoor-4127336/

Klintsons, R. (2021, April 10). *close-up-shot-of-medicines* [Image]. Pexels. https://www.pexels.com/photo/close-up-shot-of-medicines-7460060/

Krukau, Y. (2021, March 16). *pregnant-woman-sitting-on-a-yoga-ball* [Image]. Pexels.
https://www.pexels.com/photo/a-pregnant-woman-sitting-on-a-yoga-ball-7155539/

MagicBowls. (2020, January 8). *healing-music* [Image]. Pexels.
https://www.pexels.com/photo/healing-music-3544322/

Mark Hang Fung So. (2017, November 23). *Man on grass lawn* [Image]. Unsplash.com.
https://unsplash.com/photos/man-on-grass-lawn-nYtpiW06Lbg

Nature Zen. (2021, May 31). *Photo by Nature Zen on Unsplash* [Image]. Unsplash.com.
https://unsplash.com/photos/sliced-banana-and-strawberry-on-table-zF5C6-5qDxs

Pixabay. (2016, February 29). *blue-tape-measuring-on-clear-glass-square-weighing-scale* [Image]. Pexels.
https://www.pexels.com/photo/blue-tape-measuring-on-clear-glass-square-weighing-scale-53404/

Shvets, A. (2020, August 9). *aged-gray-haired-man-running-on-stadium* [Image]. Pexels.
https://www.pexels.com/photo/aged-gray-haired-man-running-on-stadium-5067669/

Smith, V. (2018, September 16). *Assorted Color Beans* [Image]. Pexels.https://www.pexels.com/photo/assorted-color-beans-in-sack-1393382/

Zomer, M. (2017, March 3). *person-holding-a-stress-ball-* [Image]. Pexels. https://www.pexels.com/photo/person-holding-a-stress-ball-339620/

Keeping it Alive

Now, you have everything you need for a successful chair yoga regimen. Congrats! The best way to pass on your new knowledge and guide others to where they can find it is by leaving a review on Amazon.

>>> Scan the QR code to leave your review.
Thank you for paying it forward. Good karma is real :)

Printed in Great Britain
by Amazon